YOUR CRITICALLY ILL CHILD

Life and Death Choices Parents Must Face

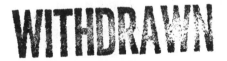

YOUR CRITICALLY ILL CHILD

Life and Death Choices Parents Must Face

By
Dr. Christopher Johnson

New Horizon Press
Far Hills, NJ

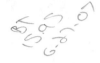

Christopher M. Johnson
Your Critically Ill Child:
Life and Death Choices Parents Must Face

Cover Design: Wendy Bass
Interior Design: Susan Sanderson

Library of Congress Control Number:

ISBN 13: 978-0-88282-284-6
ISBN 10: 0-88282-284-5
New Horizon Press

Manufactured in the U.S.A.

2009   2008   2007   2006   2005 / 5   4   3   2   1

Dedication

To my wife, Jennie, and to my children, Benjamin and Sarah, and especially to the many brave children and their families whom I have cared for over the past two decades.

Acknowledgments

This book began as a series of conversations that I have had over the years with friends and colleagues about the world of the PICU and what it can teach us. As I collected these stories and thought about their meanings, I realized that they could be as fascinating and inspiring to others as they have been to me. When it came time to write them down, John Thornton and Lisa Adams gave me very useful advice about earlier versions of the book. I thank both my agent, Anne Devlin, and my publisher, Joan Dunphy, for having high confidence in the book and in my ability to write it. I especially want to thank my editor, Barbara Cotton, for the skillful way she made the book the best that it could be.

I have been fortunate in having had several outstanding teachers who inspired me to write this book. Professor Roger Lane of Haverford College showed me that one could be both a rigorous scholar and a good storyteller, and Professor Kathleen Hable Rhodes of the Mayo Clinic College of Medicine taught me that taking excellent care of sick children requires careful listening to parents. Every parent whose child passes through the PICU knows that the true unsung heroes of the PICU are the nurses and respiratory therapists who spend many hours at sick children's bedsides; I have known and been inspired by scores of them over the years. I thank them all.

My greatest acknowledgement is to the children. This book selects only a few from the several thousand children whom I have cared for during two decades in the PICU, but all of them have unique stories and reveal crucial information which can serve as a guide when you must make life and death decisions for your critically ill child. It has been a privilege for me to care for each and every one of them.

Table of Contents

Introduction

This book is about caring for critically ill children. It details the stories of crucial decisions which had to be made in the course of treating these children in a period when they needed expert care. The book reveals many challenges and decisions that these children and their families faced when severe illness or injury unexpectedly entered their lives.

None of us are ready for events like these when they suddenly happen. However, most of us are wiser and stronger than we often think we are; we can meet these decisions, sometimes against very tall odds. It has been my privilege to watch that happen time and again.

This book is also about a new medical specialty—pediatric critical care medicine—and the place where it happens—the pediatric intensive care unit, or PICU. Practitioners of this new specialty, of which I am one, are called "pediatric intensivists," and we do our work in PICUs. Our specialty grew from hospitals' desires to bring together in one place all critically ill and injured children, whether their particular problems involved their heads or their hearts, because all of these children and their families share many common needs. Once PICUs appeared, the many medical advances in life-support technology, heart surgery, cancer therapy, and organ transplantation soon filled them with extremely sick children with complicated medical problems. Who would care for these children?

Before intensivists appeared on the medical scene, the primary physicians for children like these had generally been those who were experts in whatever a child's main problem was, such as failure of one bodily organ or another. Most critically ill or injured children, however, cannot have their problems neatly categorized and placed in an organ-specific box. For them, all of their problems overlap in constantly changing ways. Critically ill children often need the skills of organ specialists—cardiologists for their hearts, neurologists for their brains, and nephrologists for their kidneys, to list only a few—but what they especially need is a physician who has the training and the time to sit at their bedsides in the PICU and care for the whole child. What they need is a new species of doctor, one best described as a general practitioner for the extremely ill child. That doctor is the pediatric intensivist.

I believe we need a book about the pediatric intensivist and the PICU that reveals what decisions you as parents may face if your child becomes critically ill. In addition, the PICU is a fascinating place. As you will read, no television program or movie does justice to the reality of what happens there. That reality is far more complex and multi-faceted (and more intriguing and fascinating) than Hollywood script writers can imagine because the complexity of what questions to ask at such times presents challenges to children, their parents, and those of us who work in the PICU. Some of these challenges are great, some small, but few families know how they will meet them when their child needs the PICU. These stories of children, among the thousands whom I have cared for in the PICU, depict how they and their families met and surmounted these challenges. It is a book of parables. It will show you how life-and-death decisions are made, who makes them, and what information you need.

In a PICU ordinary people perform in extraordinary ways when they confront, often suddenly and unexpectedly, sick or injured children who vividly personify issues that previously seemed distant and abstract. The PICU is not a place for those with a special moral or philosophical agenda. Highly dogmatic persons do not last long in the PICU environment because what happens there every day challenges preconceived notions of right, wrong, life and death. On the other hand, if you pay attention to what goes on there, you as a parent can make wiser decisions. This is because in the PICU not only is the care intensive, but so too is the lived experience. This book will take you there to share in that experience.

This book tells personal stories of individual children and their families. Although the substance of each story took place essentially as I have written it, I have taken care to protect the privacy of these children and their families. Common decency, medical ethics, and federal law all require this. I have practiced pediatric critical care for more than twenty years in many different facilities in various parts of the country. Besides the obvious safeguard of using pseudonyms, in some cases I changed the ages and sexes of the children, and I have not identified the PICU where I cared for them. I also have changed details that might serve to identify the children. Nonetheless, I have preserved the essential truth of these stories. Although I wish all of you and your families future good health and prosperity, I am confident that the information, challenges, and decisions revealed here will serve you well if the time has or will come when one of your children becomes critically ill and you must summon all available knowledge and good judgment to make life and death decisions for him or her.

Chapter 1

Parent's Challenge: Running the PICU Marathon

Critical illness strikes children suddenly and few parents are ready when it does. We are not prepared because children are a complicated package of endearing vulnerability mixed together with resilient indestructibility. One minute we are overprotective of them and the next minute we are naively unknowing about what they are doing. The range of serious illnesses and injuries that can happen to children is terrifyingly broad. Yet in spite of this minefield of potential dangers, nearly all children escape them to become parents themselves. So although we do fear for our children, we also take comfort in the knowledge, even the expectation that things will turn out fine–and things usually do.

Sometimes, however, children need help when serious illness and accidents strike; they need parents who are knowledgeable about what experts to turn to; they need the sophisticated capabilities of the pediatric intensive care unit, the PICU.

If you have a child who may or does need expert care, the story of Robert, one child for whom I cared, shows you the wonders that our marvelous PICU technology can accomplish. His experiences also shows you that, for many children and their families, the PICU experience is like running a physical, mental, and emotional marathon. The great challenge is to complete this marathon successfully, and to do so parents must be alert and active participants in the process of finding and obtaining the best possible care when their child becomes critically ill or injured.

Robert's story will give you much vital information that I hope will benefit you and your child if the need for special care or organ donation arises. At the end of the story I have included some important points which have been contained and fleshed out in Robert's experiences.

Robert was an only child who lived in a small city with Gail, his mother. Like most children, Robert had been generally healthy during all his five years of life. Of course he had suffered a few ear-aches, experienced an occasional fever, and had a rash or two, but he had generally been an active, healthy boy. All of that changed one Sunday when Gail did not hear her son up and playing in his room as he usually did first thing in the morning. She went to check on him and saw that he was still in bed and appeared to be sleeping. When she aroused him he was groggy and he did not seem to be himself at all. He was disoriented and confused, did not answer questions coherently, and did not even seem to know where he was. Something was clearly very wrong with the boy, so Gail brought him to the emergency department of her local hospital to find out what it was. He vomited several times in the car on the way there.

The doctor in the emergency department examined Robert and found him still to be incoherent and confused. The child also did not react normally to bright lights shined in his eyes and would not obey simple commands, such as "squeeze my hand." The doctor noted a few other things besides Robert's mental confusion. For one thing, the child's skin appeared to be yellowish (jaundiced). In addition, his liver was larger than normal. In a child Robert's age, one normally feels the edge of the liver just below the ribcage on the right side of the belly. The doctor felt Robert's liver edge extending further down into his abdomen, making the organ about twice as big as it should have been. Robert also winced when the doctor pressed down to feel his liver, indicating that the organ was also abnormally tender.

Gail was confused and afraid. Yet it is important at a critical time like this for parents, in spite of their fears, to understand what the exact problem is with their child. So what *was* wrong with Robert? Several blood tests soon showed, at least in a general way, what his trouble was; his liver was inflamed, a condition called hepatitis. When most people hear the word hepatitis, they think of the common forms of that illness, typically caused by infection with a virus. By tradition, scientists have assigned these illnesses letters rather than names: hepatitis A is caused by contaminated food or water, and both hepatitis B (once called "serum hepatitis") and hepatitis C are transmitted by contaminated blood or needles or sexual contact. But there are many other viruses besides these three that can cause hepatitis, a term that really means nothing more than "inflamed liver" in Greek. Many cases of hepatitis are not even caused by viruses at all, since a wide variety of other diseases, medicines, and toxins can inflame the liver.

Most forms of hepatitis are quite mild, and often affected persons do not even know that they have anything wrong with them unless they happen to have a blood test done. Robert, however, clearly had a severe kind of hepatitis. Judging both by how sick he was and how deranged were the blood tests of his liver function, he had what we call acute fulminate hepatitis. This term is only a descriptive one. It does not really tell us anything about what was causing Robert's illness.

The doctor in Robert's home town hospital was very concerned about the child's situation, and he called me to talk over Robert's case. I shared his concern and I suggested that we transfer the child to our PICU. Robert's mother concurred. We needed to do that quickly, since it appeared likely that he would get worse, possibly far worse, before he got better. It was even possible that he would not get better; Robert's liver was failing rapidly, and severe liver damage can be permanent or even fatal. I arranged to have Robert flown from his local facility to the PICU, where I worked.

This flight was Robert's first encounter with high-tech medicine. He was to have many more during the ensuing weeks. Medical aircraft are equipped as a sort of mobile intensive care unit, and they are typically staffed by transport teams specially trained in the needs of critically ill children. Team members are in constant communication with the medical experts at their base of operations, so such teams are often able to begin sophisticated treatments even before the child reaches the PICU. Depending upon the needs of the child and the travel distance, the aircraft can either be a helicopter or a standard, fixed-wing airplane.

Robert's condition had changed by the time that he arrived in the PICU several hours later. Earlier in the morning he had been listless and confused; when he arrived in the PICU he was agitated and combative. In fact, he was hallucinating and he did not recognize his mother. I gave him a sedative medication to calm him down through the intravenous line that was running in his hand, and he dozed off in his bed. I then did some emergency blood tests, rechecking his tests that measure liver function, as well as adding some additional studies to see how bad his situation was. I also did some tests to see if Robert had inadvertently taken one of the several drugs or been exposed to one of the chemicals that can cause liver failure—he hadn't.

Robert's test results came back quickly, and they looked ominous. All of his numbers were worse than they had been only a few hours before. Robert's general condition was also looking increasingly ominous. His level of consciousness was deteriorating, meaning that he was lapsing into a coma. It was clear that I was soon going to need to use on Robert some of the high-tech medical life-support capabilities we have in the PICU. Before it all ended, my colleagues and I would need to use nearly all of them. But before you meet that technology and learn about the treatments, we need to go over a few things about what the liver is and what it does.

This then is the next point at which parents need to participate actively in their critically ill child's care; they need to gain information on the organs or parts of the body affected and how they function.

In this case the organ was the liver, which is a crucial organ for the body. It has several key functions. One of these is to remove from the bloodstream the toxic things that we may eat and drink, such as alcohol, as well as the waste products from the body's natural processes, such as occurs with the natural death and recycling of body cells. The liver is also a factory for the manufacture of most of the proteins that circulate in our bloodstream. Chief among these are the blood coagulation proteins, which are key components of the delicate system that both makes our blood clot normally in the right places and prevents it from clotting abnormally in the wrong places. A third vital function of the liver is to maintain our blood sugar in the normal range between meals. Our livers do this by steadily releasing sugar (in the form of glucose) into our bloodstreams as our other organs need it. Our hearts and brains in particular need a predictable and constant supply of glucose. A fourth important function of the liver is to make bile and to secrete this vital substance from the liver into our intestine via a tube called the bile duct. We need bile in our intestines in order to digest many fats and to absorb certain essential vitamins.

As the afternoon and early evening of Robert's first day in the PICU unfolded, he was showing all of the signs of fast developing acute liver failure. He was lapsing deeper into a coma because his liver could no longer clear body wastes and toxins from his bloodstream, particularly ammonia. As his blood concentration of ammonia rose, he became ever more deeply comatose because that is what too much ammonia does to the brain. He began to have difficulty in keeping his blood sugar level in the normal range, and he needed a constant infusion in his vein of a very high concentration of glucose to make sure that his brain and heart received enough. In addition, his liver's ability to make the all-important blood clotting proteins was becoming steadily more and more impaired. This meant that he would likely require frequent infusions into his veins of fresh plasma, which contains those proteins, to keep him from bleeding to death.

Although there are times when a child's situation is such that everyone concerned can sit around a table and talk things over, there are other times when this is not possible because events are moving too fast. Robert's situation was of the latter sort, and these situations are often the most terrifying to a child's family.

In rapidly evolving scenarios such as Robert's, I do try as much as possible to explain to families what is going on as it is happening. This sort of discussion on the fly, however, lays bare the inherent uncertainty that surrounds much of what we do in the PICU. That is, we proceed with the best information that we have at that moment, recognizing that new information may appear or events occur that send us down an entirely different treatment path. That is the reality of critical care practice. Hindsight is said to be twenty-twenty; in contrast, it is often very unclear to us in the PICU what the next minutes, hours, and days will bring as they unfold. Foremost in my mind was the fact that, although I knew that Robert's liver was failing, I did not know why.

Yet in spite of the urgency of the situation, I knew that I very much needed to take some time to talk to Gail about what was happening to her son, the boy who had never really been sick before in his life. It is very important that the doctor take the time to explain to you what is happening and what needs to occur. To do so is not merely a favor to the family; it is the doctor's responsibility. No matter what the circumstances, parents must not be shy about asking the doctor tough questions.

I sat next to Robert's bed while Gail lay in it beside him. She was long past being upset and distraught; she was numb. She had eaten little for twelve hours, subsisting on crackers and coffee from the nurse's station. She had driven hundreds of miles chasing her son in the aircraft. She was terrified by what was happening. She was also tortured by what she believed to have been her own negligence, her responsibility for Robert's condition.

Many, many parents blame themselves as Gail did for not recognizing their child's critical illness in its early stages. Blame, though, is not relevant here. What is relevant is for the parents to construct a written or oral timetable of events. Gail knew now that Robert had not sickened quite as suddenly as we had first thought. She told me that, in retrospect, Robert had not been quite himself for the previous two days. He had seemed "pale" to her, which she now realized was actually the early stages of jaundice, of liver failure. He also had taken a nap during the afternoon for several days previously, something that he had not done for years. She berated herself for not having taken Robert to the doctor then. I did not know what to tell her, other than to reassure her that she had done nothing wrong; the early signs of many serious illnesses are quite subtle. She didn't hear me—there really is no blame for that sort of pain. After I had listened to Gail for a time, something that is a crucial part of my job, I told her what I needed to do for her son.

The first thing that Robert needed was a secure way to breathe, since his ability to do that on his own was rapidly deteriorating. He needed one of the most common articles of high-tech medicine that we use in the PICU—a mechanical ventilator, a breathing machine. The machines that we use are called positive-pressure ventilators. (This distinguishes them from negative-pressure ventilators, the "iron lungs" used during the polio epidemics of the nineteen-fifties.) The first positive-pressure ventilators were primitive devices, being essentially nothing more than big bellows filled with air and oxygen that blew their contents into the child to expand the lungs. In contrast, our current machines are extremely sophisticated, with onboard electronic systems that not only breathe for the child, but also tell us a great deal about what is going on in the child's lungs. They can even sense what a child's own breathing is doing and respond appropriately.

A mechanical ventilator is high-tech, but the process of placing a child on a ventilator is decidedly low-tech, and has changed little in forty years. The first step is endotracheal intubation, inserting the breathing tube that will connect the child's lungs to the ventilator. This is not easy. If I were simply to push the endotracheal tube into Robert's mouth and down into his throat, it would most likely not go where it needs to go–the windpipe, or trachea. Rather, it would pass down into his esophagus, the swallowing tube leading to the stomach. Unrecognized placement of an endotracheal tube in the esophagus, rather than in the trachea, is one of the most dreaded catastrophes that can occur during intubation.

To get the endotracheal tube in the right place, I use a device called a laryngoscope. This is nothing more than a curved metal blade with a light on the end so that I can see into the trachea. With the child lying on his back, I first use my left hand to place the smooth-edged blade in the child's mouth and with it move the tongue out of the way. I next manipulate the tip of the blade to lift up the epiglottis, a flap of tissue that protects the opening to the trachea by preventing food from getting into the airway when the child swallows. When all goes well, I can do this maneuver in nearly one quick motion, thereby exposing the opening to the child's trachea. Once I can see where to put the breathing tube, I then use my right hand to pass its tip between the child's vocal cords and on down into the trachea. I then remove the laryngoscope from the child's mouth and connect the end of the breathing tube, which now protrudes from the mouth by a few inches, to a hand ventilator, a simple device with a soft bag full of oxygen that I squeeze to force air through the tube and down into the child's lungs. This tells me that the tube is in the right place.

Being intubated is extremely uncomfortable. Indeed, it is essentially impossible to manage to do it on a fully conscious child, although some adults can be intubated using only light sedation and some medication to numb the tissues in the back of the throat so that the tube will not cause them to gag. In children, particularly very young ones who cannot comprehend what is happening to them, we routinely use medications to put the child completely asleep and relax the muscles. These drugs carry significant risks. In fact, potential disaster lurks at every step of the intubation process. In Robert's case, however, everything went well. Once I had placed his breathing tube in the right place, I connected it to a mechanical ventilator and adjusted the settings on the machine to give him a satisfactory breathing pattern.

Once Robert was safely on the ventilator, I attended to some of the other life-support and monitoring equipment that he needed. Since he was in a deep coma, he could not urinate normally and needed a plastic tube, a Foley catheter, put into his bladder to drain urine. He also needed yet another plastic tube, a nasogastric tube, passed through one of his nostrils and down into his stomach and connected to a suction device, since without this his stomach and intestines would become bloated with air. Later on in a child's course we often use these tubes to give liquid feedings into the stomach.

I also needed the nasogastric tube to see if Robert was bleeding into his stomach, since this is a common problem in patients with liver failure. In fact, he was bleeding profusely from the lining of his stomach. I knew this because after I had passed the tube through his nose I put a syringe on the end and pulled back on the plunger; nearly a cup of fresh blood came back into the syringe. This was serious and required immediate treatment with fresh plasma, which contains the needed blood clotting proteins that his liver was not making. I also gave him a drug that blocked his stomach's ability to produce acid. This medicine helps to decrease the bleeding by reducing the irritation that stomach acid causes to the stomach lining.

I next needed to place two kinds of long, thin tubes, or catheters, in Robert's blood vessels. Robert needed these "lines" to monitor minute to minute what was happening with the function of his cardiovascular system and with the amount of oxygen in his blood. The lines also allowed me to give Robert all of the many medications, blood transfusions, and plasma transfusions that he would need. Additionally, they allowed me to take blood samples from Robert without the need for additional needle sticks. For one of these lines I used the femoral vein in his groin as an entry point to pass the ten inch long catheter into his inferior vena cava, the large vein in the center of his body. For the other I used his radial artery, the artery in his wrist where one normally feels the pulse.

Whether or not parents should be present when these things are done to their children is a subject of some controversy. My own practice is to try to gauge how the parents might react and I then often give them the option of staying or not. Gail had waited outside in the parents' lounge while I intubated Robert and placed his various tubes and lines.

Over the past decade, I have noticed that more and more parents choose to stay with their children. If they wish to stay and see the procedure, however, it is important for the physician again to explain everything that is happening. I have found it is also important to have the parents sit down, since I have had more than a few parents get queasy or even faint to the floor when they see such procedures being done to their child. On the other hand, some parents have told me that their imagination of what their child might be going through was worse than seeing the real thing, so they were glad that they had stayed. Their presence may help their child to adjust as much as possible. If you feel you need or want to be present, make your wishes known, even if your child's doctor does not ask you about it.

Gail felt she would be too nervous and frightened to offer reassurance while I did these procedures. She waited outside and when she got back I met her at the door to prepare her for what she would see. If your child is to receive all of the treatments as those given to Robert, you will be confronted by the sight of plastic tubes coming out of his or her nose, mouth, groin, and wrist, with wads of tape holding all of these things in place. The chest will be plastered with electrodes that go to the heart and breathing monitors. Eyes will appear slimy due to the artificial tears that we use to protect the eyes of patients who are too sedated to blink normally. There will be a lighted probe on the finger to tell us the blood oxygen level. The ventilator hisses periodically and the room will be filled with strange beeps and alarms. All of this technology is familiar to PICU workers, but no one else is really ready for a sight like that. Yet within a few hours Gail, like most parents in this situation, mustered her courage and found the strength to look past the tubes and lines to see her son lying in the bed. We are truly an adaptable species.

Once I had done all of the things that Robert needed immediately, I turned my attention to the most important issue, which was what had happened to Robert, and what was wrong with his liver. To find that out I needed help from my expert colleagues, particularly those who specialize in liver disease. Since the liver is primarily a part of the digestive system, the experts in liver diseases are those physicians with special training in digestive diseases, the pediatric gastroenterologists. One came to see Robert the afternoon that the child arrived in the PICU. He went over all of the tests that we had done thus far, examined Robert, and spoke with Gail. Although he could not be sure, the gastroenterologist suspected that Robert had a severe viral infection that had attacked his liver. The reason that he could not know for sure is because diagnosing viral infections is not easy. Viruses grow very slowly in the laboratory, if they grow at all. Instead of growing the virus, we often diagnose viral infections indirectly by testing the blood for evidence that the child has been exposed to a virus recently. These tests, however, also take time and they are not universally reliable.

The best way for us to determine what was wrong with Robert's liver would be to get a sample of the liver itself, a biopsy, both to look for viruses and to see under the microscope what was happening to the liver cells. Liver biopsies can be done in several ways. The most common and easiest way is to pass a long, thin needle through the skin and into the liver. The needle has a device inside of it to take a small piece of liver and hold it securely while the needle is removed. Although the piece is small, it is usually large enough for our purposes. Another way to biopsy the liver is for a surgeon to do an operation called a laparotomy—open the child's abdomen and cut out a wedge of liver tissue for study. A variant of laparotomy is called laparoscopy, in which the surgeon makes a smaller incision near the liver and through it inserts into the abdominal cavity a laparoscope, a device about the size of one's finger, and with this snips off a piece of the liver. Of these, the needle biopsy is the least complicated and safest to perform.

Robert, however, was too sick to have any of these procedures. He was having too much trouble with bleeding; his liver, which normally makes the proteins that cause our blood to clot, was too diseased to make those needed clotting proteins. The liver is prone to bleed even under normal circumstances when its surface is nicked or poked. Doing a biopsy on a patient who is already bleeding is highly risky. It is true that we could have given Robert large doses of clotting proteins in the form of blood plasma, a procedure which would have transiently improved his clotting situation and briefly lowered the risk of bleeding. We sometimes do that. However, the gastroenterologist told Gail that to care for Robert at that moment we did not need the information that the biopsy would give us, so doing the procedure then was not worth the risk. This is a key point for parents: Nothing in the PICU is risk-free, so when a doctor wants to do a procedure on your child, always ask if the risk of doing it outweighs the risk of *not* doing it.

While the gastroenterologist was completing his evaluation, Robert was getting worse. I was already giving him plasma to reduce his bleeding problems, high doses of glucose to keep his blood sugar in the acceptable range, and several medications designed to reduce the amount of ammonia in his blood. But despite my efforts, Robert's coma was getting deeper. I could tell this by testing his brain function using some decidedly low-tech procedures: shining a light in his eyes to test what his pupils did, brushing a wisp of cotton on the surface of his eye to see if he blinked, pinching him to see if he moved, and touching his tongue with a wooden stick to see if he gagged. I also did a much more sophisticated test, a computerized tomographic scan (CT scan) of his brain. This test, which is a kind of x-ray of the brain, showed that Robert's brain was swelling, a condition called cerebral edema. If it continued unabated, it would kill him.

Cerebral edema in children with liver failure is a well known problem. The main reason that it is potentially so deadly is because of the brain's anatomy. The brain is completely enclosed in the hard case of the skull, armor which protects it from blows to the head. But this means that if the brain begins to swell, there is no place for the swelling tissue to go; it pushes against the constricting bony cage of the skull in a way that can block blood from flowing into the brain. The concept is simple: for blood to get into the brain, the pressure inside of the skull must be less than the blood pressure outside of the skull because blood, like any fluid, will not flow uphill. And if the brain does not get a constant supply of blood, the brain cells will be severely damaged. Even worse, if the pressure inside of the skull gets too high, the brain itself may be forced out of the bottom of the skull, a catastrophe called brain herniation. It is always fatal, and it is a common cause of death for patients with severe cerebral edema.

Unfortunately, our treatments for severe brain swelling of the sort that Robert had are meager. We can give one of several medications that help to draw the fluid from the brain, and I gave him one of those. It seemed to help for the moment. Extreme treatments, such as removing part of the skull to relieve pressure on the brain, have been tried by some physicians in such situations. Although doing this makes intuitive sense, my own experience in the past with that sort of intervention has not been good. Still, I did ask a neurosurgeon to evaluate Robert to see if he had any suggestions to offer; he did not think that any brain surgery would help. Moreover, Robert's bleeding problem from his liver failure was so severe that the neurosurgeon also did not even want to take the risk of placing in the brain a monitoring device that we often use to guide our therapy, a device which tells us exactly what the pressure is inside the child's brain.

So, only twenty-four hours after Robert arrived in the PICU, we had to tell his mother he was on the edge of death. What could be done? The only thing that could save Robert was to find him a new liver–to get him a liver transplant. We needed to take his destroyed liver out and give him a new one. Unfortunately, we had little time to find Robert a new liver because the experts estimated that we had only a few days, perhaps a week at most, before Robert would die of liver failure.

Organ transplantation in children is now somewhat common. Improved surgical techniques, better ways of preserving organs for transplant, and better regional and national organization of organ transplant networks have made organ transplants more frequent. Probably the single most important advance in organ transplantation technology has been the discovery of a family of powerful drugs—the first of which is cyclosporine—to prevent the organ recipient from rejecting the newly transplanted organ.

But as a parent, if your child needs such a transplant, you need to get all the information you can on how, where, when, and why. Quiz the experts called in to consult on your child's case, but do some investigating on your own as well. Carefully used, the internet is an excellent information source. Look for reliable sites, such as those sponsored by major children's hospitals. The internet is also an excellent place to look for support groups made up of parents who are going or have gone through the same ordeal as you.

Some organ transplants are done by having a living person donate the tissue. This is now the case for over half of kidney transplants. Liver transplants, however, are only rarely done using living donors, and the very notion is a controversial one because, whereas donating a kidney puts the donor at little risk from the surgery that removes the organ, there are substantial risks to donating part of one's liver. Some donors of liver tissue have even died. For this reason liver transplants are generally done using all or part of a liver donated by someone who has died. Even though there are many more patients waiting on transplant lists than there are organs for them, there is a priority system such that patients in dire need move to the top of the list, and Robert certainly qualified for top priority. Early in his second PICU day, our surgeons listed Robert in the national transplant database requesting a liver for him.

Meanwhile, Robert's condition was steadily worsening. His blood ammonia level was difficult to control, his blood sugar levels were dangerously low in spite of giving him the maximum amount of sugar in his veins that we could, and his bleeding problems were so bad that he was requiring a near constant infusion of blood plasma. To make matters worse, Robert's kidneys were starting to fail as well. There was nothing intrinsically wrong with his kidneys, but children in liver failure often develop this additional problem. Hardly an hour passed in which I did not need to intervene in some way to keep Robert alive because he had life-threatening derangements in his blood oxygen, his blood acid, his blood potassium, his blood sugar, or the amount of water in his circulation. His brain continued to swell. He had several seizures, or convulsions. He was oozing blood from his nose, his mouth, his lungs, his intestines, and the holes in his skin where needles had been.

Robert's mother had been at her son's bedside this entire time. Like many parents in a situation like this, she was terrified to leave her child for fear that he would die when she was gone, even if only to take a shower or get a meal. Gail was also dealing with a problem that many parents find difficult when their child is critically ill in a large PICU–an overabundance of doctors. It is good to have so many experts to help and give advice, but the inevitable conflicting interpretations of what is going on and what to do can be unbearable for parents. Nevertheless, you must steel yourself to hear it, ask questions and get information. (You will read more about this in the next chapter.)

What I and most of my intensivist colleagues strive to do to alleviate this problem is to be there at the bedside when each of the many experts speak with a child's family. In Robert's case, this list included the gastroenterologist, the transplant surgeon, the hematologist (an expert in bleeding problems), and the nephrologist (an expert in the kidney). After each of these consultants had weighed in with their opinions, I interpreted for Gail what they meant and how it all fitted together in the big picture of Robert's situation.

Pediatric critical care is in many ways like an old-fashioned general practice, because, like the old-time general practitioners, I and my colleagues must deal with all aspects of a child's problem. And minding the high-tech machinery is only one of those aspects. In fact, for some children in the PICU, the technology plays only a minor role in their care. This is the paradox of intensive care: nowhere is humanistic medical practice more important than in medicine's most technologically sophisticated setting. Robert's situation shows the truth of this statement.

Gail was progressively falling apart under the strain. She was a twenty-two year old single mother, had no other children, and had no close family members living nearby. Robert's father was not an active parent, and she had not spoken with him for several years. Gail's own mother lived far away in another state, although she was planning to come to be with Gail as soon as she could. Gail was suffering from a constellation of problems we commonly see in families whose children are in the PICU, and which we lump together under the term "PICUitis." The cause is a combination of stress, fatigue, fear, and information overload. Chronic sleep deprivation, not eating enough, and worrying take a fearful toll on the body. I usually see families get "PICUitis" beginning on about the second day of their child's stay in the PICU, particularly if the child's situation is one of constant crisis such as was Robert's. Gail was developing a severe case.

Most PICU staffers do what they can to get families to eat, sleep, and shower, but most parents find it difficult to leave their child's bedside. Remember, if you are to be the best help to your child you must take care of yourself, eat adequately, and get sufficient rest. In our PICU, like most, there are no set visiting hours, and parents are encouraged to come and go as they wish. This policy is a good one, but sometimes it is difficult for parents to accept that we do not expect them to be there all of the time. Gail, like many parents, was feeling that she needed to be there constantly. If your child is in such a unit, know that parents often feel helpless in the high-tech world of the PICU. Yet even if you are only holding your child's hand, only you can really give that sort of comfort to your child. Like Gail, many parents feel some responsibility for their child's illness, and this makes it even more difficult for them to take a break from watching over their child. It is important, though, to get away, if only for a short time, to revitalize and help you cope in a very difficult time.

If you find yourself in Gail's situation, you need to cope with information overload because you will be bombarded with information. Some of this will come from doctors, nurses, and other PICU staff. You may glean some of it from sources as varied as the monitor screens on the equipment in your child's room and overheard conversations. Understand that, although this information can be confusing, it is overall a good thing.

Some parents sit at their child's bedside and surf the internet on their laptop computers, searching for any information that they can find on their child's condition. The relationship between physicians and patients has been evolving over the past decades from the paternalistic, "doctor knows best" view of fifty years ago, that patients should be told little about their child's case, to a viewpoint that stresses parent's involvement, even control, of all decisions about treatment. Although this can be taken too far—doctors must not use it to shirk their responsibilities—this is overall a healthy trend.

I believe parents of children in the PICU need to be told all aspects of what is going on with their children. Parents, however, still need to make decisions with clear guidance from physicians. That guidance comes from the physician taking the time to sit down with parents at the bedside, not by standing near the door, glancing at the clock. Insist on your physician giving you all relevant information about your child. If necessary, request a scheduled time to meet. No matter how hectic the situation, parents of a critically ill child should feel as if they have my complete attention.

The next time that I sat down with Gail in her son's room we talked about many things: liver transplants, what the future might bring, when her mother might come, whether she should continue to try to locate Robert's father. I gave Gail the advice of which I earlier spoke: having a critically ill child in the PICU is like running a marathon, and she needed to find a way to pace herself, to hold some emotional capital in reserve to spend during the coming days and weeks.

This is advice I strongly pass on to you. Gail also felt an ambivalence that I have encountered before, and I want to convey it to you. Parents of children waiting for a transplant realize that for their child to live, another person must die. So even though they hope every day for the transplant to happen, they wrestle with the sad feeling that this may amount to wishing for someone else's death. This situation is especially poignant when a child dies in the PICU whose parents wish to donate their child's organs, there is another child waiting in the PICU for an organ, and the two are a match. In one case where I saw this happen, although the PICU staff tried very hard to be circumspect about what was going on, the respective families found out. The bond that developed between those families was one of the most profoundly moving things that I have ever seen.

As events turned out, Robert was extremely lucky. He spent about a day and a half waiting on the transplant list before an appropriately matched liver became available for him in another city. Our transplant group quickly assembled a team to travel by jet to that city to get the liver while we in the PICU readied Robert for the operation as best we could, although he continued to be quite unstable. But although he was in poor shape to have a major operation, we had no alternative.

To save precious time, the surgeon typically begins the operation on the recipient before the donor liver actually arrives in the operating room. However, the surgeon does not proceed to the point of no return, that of removing the child's old liver, until the new liver is actually there and verified as clearly an appropriate one for the child. The time that the operation actually takes to complete varies a great deal. Often the most difficult part for the surgeon is removing the old, diseased liver, because it may be scarred tightly into the child's abdominal cavity. But Robert's old liver, which was by then shrunken down to a fraction of its healthy size, was easy for the surgeon to remove. He placed Robert's new liver where the old one was, connected the donor blood vessels to Robert's vessels, and sewed Robert's new bile duct into his intestine. When all of this was finished, Robert returned to the PICU, where Gail was waiting anxiously in his room with Robert's grandmother, who had just arrived.

Meanwhile, Robert was showing something that we occasionally see in children who receive a liver transplant; within minutes of having his new liver connected to his system, Robert began to get better. By the time he got back to the PICU from the operating room his blood chemistries and blood sugars were already much improved. By the next day his blood clotting problems had markedly improved. In fact, one of our great concerns just after liver transplant often is that a child's blood clotting problems will have improved so much that the child's system clots off the vessels leading to the new liver. We do various things to lesson the chances of this happening, but it is always a risk. Robert had no such problems and by two days after his transplant operation he had awakened to the extent that I was able to take him off the mechanical ventilator machine. Later that day he smiled and spoke to his mother for the first time since that initial morning in the emergency department. His new liver was working just fine.

Over the next few days Robert continued to get steadily better. We were able to take some of his lines out and even to let him start drinking sips of juice. Everything was going great until the morning six days after his transplant, when he had a fever. Fever is particularly concerning in children who, like Robert, are taking medications that suppress the immune system. These medicines are what allow us to do transplants, since they suppress the recipient's immune system just enough so that it will not attack and reject the new organ, but not so much that the recipient's immune system will be totally unable to do its job of fighting off infections. But achieving this balance is tricky in practice, and children in Robert's situation are especially vulnerable to all sorts of infections.

I started some tests to see if the fever might be caused by bacteria in his bloodstream, and started Robert on several antibiotics while we waited for the test results to come back. By the next day the tests showed that Robert did have a serious infection in his bloodstream. He also was rapidly getting sicker. His fevers were higher, his blood pressure was dropping below normal, his kidneys began to fail, and he was getting short of breath and needing oxygen to breathe. By the next day, he was again critically ill. I had to put him back on a mechanical ventilator because his lungs had rapidly filled with fluid. I also had to connect him to yet another high-tech machine–an artificial kidney machine–because his own kidneys were not working. He needed infusions of several potent medicines in his veins in order to keep his heart working adequately. After all that Robert and Gail had been through, what had happened to the poor child now?

Unfortunately and unluckily for Robert, he had developed a condition that goes by several names, but which is most commonly called sepsis or septic shock. Sepsis is best described as an out-of-control inflammatory state that affects the entire body. There are many things that can trigger the disorder, but bacteria in the bloodstream, such as Robert had, is the most common of these. Once the condition is fully underway in a child, it can cause derangements of most of the organs of the body, two of the most important of which are the lungs and the kidneys. This is what happened to Robert, and it made him as sick as he had been before his liver transplant. And as was the case with his initial liver failure, sepsis is a frequent killer. So, in a sense, we were back to square one.

This turn of events was particularly cruel for Gail, who had sat next to her son's bedside for a week as he had endured all of this. If your child is in the PICU you, like Gail, will be required to valiantly walk the emotional tightrope that the PICU demands of parents: hoping for the best while preparing for the worst.

Gail had pasted pictures on the wall of Robert's room to show all of the doctors and nurses, and to remind herself, what her child looked like before he was sick. She had gone from almost never sleeping during the time of his transplant, to dozing in the recliner chair in Robert's room. She did this partly because she was still sleep-deprived from her son's and her ordeal, but it seemed to me that she also did this as a way to defend her psyche from the surrounding chaos; if she were asleep, no one could approach her with yet more bad news about her son.

Parents need to be prepared that seeing their children's appearance in intensive care will be a shock. However, it is one which must be borne and many parents courageously handle this extremely difficult time with grace and fortitude. Robert's appearance was frightful. He was once again comatose, this time in part from the sedative medications that we had to give him to enable us to use the ventilator machine. Once again he had plastic tubes and lines coming out of everywhere in his body. His skin was still yellow from the jaundice and was covered with old bruises. But now his whole body was bloated, his skin shiny and stretched because his kidney failure was causing his body to retain too much fluid. His face was particularly affected by this, and his eyelids were swollen shut. Some of the fluid oozed out through the edges of the huge incisions on his abdomen from his liver transplant and from places in his body where lines and needles had previously broken his skin.

Robert was also connected to machinery that was even more complicated and sophisticated than he had required before his liver transplant. He was tethered via large catheters into his blood vessels to a complicated apparatus that helped his kidneys try to deal with all of the excess fluid and waste products in his body. His mechanical ventilator was different from the standard one that we had used before his transplant. Now his lungs were so stiff with fluid that he required a breathing machine that we call a high-frequency oscillator. Unlike his previous ventilator, which hissed quietly in the corner as it breathed for him, an oscillator sounds like an unbalanced washing machine on spin cycle. It is so loud that what most parents notice when it is finally not needed is the eerie silence that follows, so accustomed have they gotten to the noise. In Robert's case, the settings on his oscillator were turned up nearly as high as they could go, and still we were only barely getting sufficient oxygen into his bloodstream to keep him alive.

Robert endured this condition for over a week, living quite literally on the threshold of dying. Hardly a six hour period passed without some new crisis with his blood chemistries, or wild swings in his blood oxygen levels, or some issue with his life support machinery that needed adjustment. His need for constant infusions into his veins of medicines to support his heart was so marked that any interruption in these infusions, even for the few seconds that it took to make necessary changes in the pumps, caused his blood pressure to plummet. But in spite of it all, his new liver continued to work. That was the ray of hope for his mother and those who took care of him; we knew that if we could get him through these sepsis-related problems, we still had a chance to cure him. Insist on being made aware if your child is going through such complications and keep a record of who is caring for him or her—and know there is still hope. I expressed that hope to Gail every day. If you ever find yourself in a situation like Gail's, the key question to ask the doctor is: "Is there still hope?"

And then Robert began to get better–not all of a sudden, but gradually and very steadily day by day. We were not really aware at the moment that any corners had been turned or thresholds crossed. It was only by looking back that his steady improvement became clear to all of us. The first small step on Robert's path to recovery was that he quit being the center of attention in the PICU. He no longer had the dubious honor of being the sickest child in the PICU, and I could go and get dinner or coffee without the expectation that my beeper would summon me back to his bedside with some new crisis. Gail could leave the hospital for a few hours without fearing catastrophe. After a few more days, she even could spend the night sleeping in a real bed outside of the hospital.

Robert's recovery then began to accelerate. His kidneys improved to the point that we could remove him from the artificial machinery, and his swelling resolved so that he looked like himself again. His new liver cleared the yellow jaundice from his skin. The wounds from his transplant surgery healed. His lungs were healing, too, and I was next able to take him off the oscillator ventilator machine and place him on a standard ventilator. He was still deeply sedated with medications, however, so we could not tell if his ordeal had caused him any permanent injury to his brain, as sometimes happens. As Robert's lungs improved further, we began the steps to take him off the breathing machine, a process that has been aptly termed "liberation from mechanical ventilation."

Over the next few days we reduced the doses of Robert's sedative medications and turned down the settings on his ventilator. This had the effect of waking him up and asking him to take over more and more of his own breathing; it weaned him from the machine. With a patient such as Robert, we often do not know how this weaning process will go until we try. Some children are so weak from their illness (particularly if they have needed a ventilator for many days) that they will not be strong enough to breathe completely on their own. These children continue to need prolonged help from the machine for some or all of the day until they build their strength back. Other children take a very long time for the sedative medications to wash out of their systems and they are too unaware to breathe normally until that happens.

In Robert's case, the weaning process took about five days. At the end of that time I pulled the endotracheal tube from his mouth and he breathed fine on his own. He was weak and groggy, but he clearly recognized his mother, who was at last able to hold him again without a nest of tubes, lines, and wires getting in the way. By the next day Robert was again drinking some clear fluids like juice, and by the day after that he was actually taking a more regular diet without problems. He got out of bed and sat in a chair with Gail for a few hours. By then the only medications that he was taking were those that he needed to prevent his body from rejecting his transplanted liver. He was safely back.

Robert owes his life to high-tech medical machinery, procedures, and medicines, and his story shows what the PICU and its marvelous wonders can do. Mere hours after he first got sick, an aircraft staffed by a specially trained pediatric transport team flew Robert to the PICU. There complicated life-support machinery and medicines kept him alive while he was waiting for his liver transplant, a procedure which required the skills of dozens of highly trained individuals. His subsequent episode of septic shock would have killed him were it not for additional sophisticated machines and the skills of still dozens more of highly trained doctors, nurses, and technicians. Twelve years later he was in high school, complaining that his mother would not let him drive their car to the big city by himself. She thought that it was too dangerous.

Robert's story also encapsulates several of the principal challenges for parents of children in the PICU. Chief among these challenges are understanding just what the PICU is and what can and cannot be done there. Yet it takes more than just this understanding for families to successfully run the physical and emotional marathon that PICU care can be for them and their children; it takes active parents who question, get information, and help make crucial decisions for and about their critically ill child with their child's doctors and other caregivers. It also takes patience and faith. The rest of the stories and information in this book will show you why that is so and give you crucial advice if your child needs PICU care.

CRUCIAL ADVICE FOR PARENTS

Be alert and active in finding and gaining the best possible care in terms of medical specialists and hospitals to care for your critically ill child.

Ascertain from experts just what the exact problem or condition is in terms that your will understand.

Research your child's problem on your own so that you understand the function of the parts of the body and the organs affected.

Keep a record of who is caring for your child, what is being done, and why.

Insist that your doctor take the time to discuss with you all important information.

Take care of yourself so that you can properly care for your child; get adequate rest and nutrition.

Chapter 2

How the PICU Works

Parents need to prepare themselves before emergencies happen if they are to get the best care for their children. One way to do this is to understand how PICUs evolved and how they work. This chapter will give you a general look at the goings-on in a typical PICU, but you need to check the one nearest you to find out what facilities are available since not all PICUs are equipped to handle all cases.

Hospitals began to establish specialized PICU units when they realized that critically ill and injured children and their families have many things in common, whether a child's particular problem involves his heart or his head. Once PICUs began to appear, nurses and physicians who were interested in caring for critically ill children increasingly developed the unique and special skills needed to provide that care. The formal specialty of pediatric critical care was not really planned in advance by anyone. Instead, like PICUs, it began and grew in response to children's needs. The first pediatric intensivists learned their trade on the job. These pioneers of our field then came together to formalize what it meant to be a specialist in the field, what training and experience were needed to practice pediatric critical care. Even though PICUs were originally organized more for geographic than medical reasons, the result has been that both the art and the science of pediatric critical care medicine have flourished. The most important result has been better care for critically ill children and their families.

The PICU is a marvelous and sophisticated place. It is also a place that parents and families can find confusing and complicated, and sometimes even incomprehensible. Some of the confusion is inevitable because sometimes even the doctors are unsure about what is happening with a particular child. This is part of the reality of critical care medicine. This also means that, for many families with a child in the PICU, it is a major challenge simply to grasp what is going on around them. The inherent chaos of the PICU can be a frustrating and even frightening experience for parents.

Coping with this fear and frustration is one of the major challenges of having a child in the PICU. The whole place can appear similar to the way that the pioneering psychologist William James described the inner world of an infant: "one big blooming, buzzing confusion." James described the situation one way. A professor of mine put it another way: his favorite saying was that "things are complicated." This chapter tells the story of a child whose PICU stay was complicated in the extreme. Reading his story will help prepare you for some of the confusion and inherent uncertainty of having a child in the PICU by letting you experience that confusion alongside me as it unfolds. This chapter will also help you understand the various medical specialists' roles in such a unit.

Ronnie was a fifteen-year-old boy who came to the PICU late one June evening. His case well illustrates some of the vital care aspects you may need to call on for your child. The details of what exactly had happened to him were unclear to us for many days, and that uncertainty was part of our problem in figuring out how to care for him. Two hikers found him lying unconscious in the woods on a summer evening. He was sprawled at the base of a large rock formation, and it appeared to the hikers that he had fallen from them, a vertical distance of about twenty feet. When the hikers tried to arouse Ronnie by speaking to him, the child moaned but did not awaken. While one of the hikers went to get help (this all happened at a time before the near universal presence of cellular telephones in pocket or pack), the other stayed with Ronnie.

This hiker who remained with Ronnie was a volunteer fireman with some training in how to care for injured persons, and he noted several things that he clearly described to me later. He felt Ronnie's pulse at the child's wrist; although the pulse felt rapid and weak, it was at least definitely present. The hiker also checked how Ronnie was breathing; even though the child's breaths were shallow, they, too, at least were present. The child did not have dusky lips or other evidence of inadequate breathing. The fireman noted that Ronnie had several injuries. These included a fair-sized bruise on the child's forehead, a mildly swollen wrist, and a quite large area of swelling over the thigh; Ronnie moaned when the hiker squeezed either the child's wrist or thigh. The hiker then remembered (correctly) from his fire rescue training that hypothermia, or severe cold stress, can be deadly to injured persons. Even though it was summer, nighttime in that part of the country can be quite chilly, so the hiker took off his coat to cover Ronnie and added the spare clothing that he had in his pack. He then waited for his partner to return with help.

Ronnie's journey to the PICU took nearly twelve hours. A local rescue team of volunteers and a paramedic returned to the scene with the first hiker. The paramedic began an intravenous line to give the child some needed fluid and did a more complete examination than the hiker's useful, but necessarily cursory once-over. It appeared to the paramedic that Ronnie's wrist and leg were both broken, and he placed splints and padding around both of these. The paramedic took Ronnie's temperature, and noted that it was several degrees below normal in spite of the extra clothing covering him. The rescue team then carried Ronnie by litter five miles to an ambulance parked at the nearest road. From there he went to the emergency department of the nearby small hospital, was stabilized there, and then sent on to my PICU. During the trip Ronnie still had not awakened, but he continued to breathe sufficiently well to get enough oxygen into his bloodstream. Even so, the rescue team gave him extra oxygen from a portable tank just to be safe. He continued to respond to being moved by moaning or even mumbling a few incoherent words. By the time that he reached his local hospital the intravenous fluids had improved his circulation substantially, and the warm blankets had restored his temperature to normal.

Once Ronnie arrived in our emergency department, the physicians there examined him and did a battery of tests to discover the extent of his injuries. As the paramedic had suspected, these injuries included a broken wrist and a broken femur, the large bone in the upper leg. Broken femurs often cause significant bleeding into the tissues around the bone, and

Ronnie's blood counts showed that he had indeed lost a great deal of blood. A CT scan of Ronnie's brain showed that the child had struck his head and cracked his skull, presumably on a rock when he fell, and that this had caused a small bruise on the surface of Ronnie's brain beneath the skull fracture. Of even more concern than the bleeding was the fact that Ronnie's brain also had swollen mildly—cerebral edema, the same sort of problem that Robert, the child in the last chapter, had experienced. Fortunately for Ronnie, his brain swelling was much less severe than Robert's had been, but as was the case with Robert, the swelling made Ronnie progressively less aware of his surroundings; he was lapsing into a coma. Within an hour after arriving in the emergency department, Ronnie's coma was sufficiently deep that he was no longer breathing reliably on his own, so the doctors there had to intubate the child's airway with a breathing tube and place him on a mechanical ventilator.

Ronnie was critically ill when he reached the PICU, but at that point everyone involved in his care thought that we knew what was going on with the child, what his list of serious problems contained. By that time he had been examined and evaluated by several different kinds of physicians: a neurosurgeon had seen him for his skull fracture and his brain swelling, an orthopedic surgeon had evaluated and splinted his broken bones, and a general surgeon had looked him over to find any evidence of internal injuries caused by the fall that we all assumed that he had experienced. Even though patients who have fallen like Ronnie often suffer injuries to their abdominal organs, such as their livers and spleens, in this respect at least Ronnie had been lucky; none of this had happened to him. So when he arrived in the PICU we thought that we were pretty sure what we were dealing with: a child who had suffered a closed head injury causing mild brain swelling and resultant coma, and who also had a couple of broken bones that had caused him to lose quite a bit of blood. This is pretty standard stuff for the PICU staff.

That was Ronnie's assumed medical situation. His social situation was much murkier because, not only had we no certain report of what had happened to him, we did not know very much about him. In fact, we were not able to talk to any of his family until many hours after Ronnie had arrived in the PICU. Late that night Ronnie's grandparents arrived in the PICU, and they were able to tell us at least part of the story. Ronnie had been staying with them for several weeks while the child's parents were away on an extended trip in a very remote region of another state. Two days previously, he had had a fight with his grandparents and had run away, taking some food and camping equipment with him. When his grandparents realized that he was gone, they called the local sheriff's office to get help in finding Ronnie, although they had no idea in what direction he had gone. After the search-and-rescue team brought Ronnie out of the woods, the sheriff made the connection with his missing-child report, called Ronnie's grandparents, and they came to the local hospital and identified Ronnie before he was transported to our PICU. His grandparents had also tried to locate Ronnie's parents, but they had thus far been unsuccessful and were unsure as to how long that it might take to find them.

In the beginning we had no medical history on Ronnie. Luckily, Ronnie's grandparents were able to tell us quite a bit more about him. In that sense they cleared up some of our confusion about his case, but they also added to it. His grandparents said Ronnie was a child with several chronic health-related problems, at least one of which may have contributed to his present injuries. Ronnie had epilepsy, a condition that caused him to have occasional generalized convulsions, termed grand mal seizures. Ronnie had suffered from these seizures since he was six years old. His convulsions tended to occur every month or so, even though he took medicine every day intended to prevent them. His grandparents said that, although the medication did not completely prevent the seizures, without any medication Ronnie had seizures nearly every day, and they were much more severe than those that he experienced while taking medicine. They knew that Ronnie had not been taking his medicine for the past several days at least, because he had not taken his medicine with him when he ran away. His grandparents also suspected that Ronnie had not been taking his medicine regularly for some time; they had brought with them the bottle that contained his medication, and after counting the pills it appeared as if there were too many in the bottle.

Ronnie's situation demonstrates how important it is for parents to keep a medical record for their child, particularly if he or she has major medical problems or takes medications regularly. Keep a copy of this record in a safe place and give it to anyone who is taking care of your children while you are away. This is particularly important if your child is admitted to a PICU.

Ronnie had other problems besides the seizures. His doctor had diagnosed him with what is usually called "attention deficit hyperactivity disorder," or ADHD, because Ronnie was having progressively worse troubles at school and had been held back a grade the previous year. He was impulsive and sometimes difficult to control. This was not the first time that he had run away from home, and he had been picked up by the police several times for minor infractions. In the past he had taken various medications intended to control his ADHD, but none of them had seemed to his parents to help Ronnie's behavior very much, so they had stopped giving them to him several months previously. His parents even wondered if the medications were making his seizures worse. Ronnie's behavior had indeed become much worse over the past several months and he had become much more difficult for his parents to manage. They worried that he might be taking illicit drugs. In fact, the reason that Ronnie's parents were gone on the extended trip was to give both them and Ronnie a break from all of the chronic conflict within the family.

We still were confused about what had happened to Ronnie, but this new information from his grandparents, plus some test results, gave us a few clues as to how he might have been injured. We tested his blood for the presence of his anti-seizure medication; there was none there, so this confirmed that he had not been taking any of it at least for the past forty-eight hours or so. As is routine in cases like Ronnie's, that is of a patient found with an altered mental state, we also did tests of his blood and his urine to see if he had evidence of any illicit drugs in his system, and his urine tested positive for marijuana. This drug persists in the urine for many days after a person smokes or eats it, so we could not be sure when Ronnie had taken it. His parents had told his grandparents that they had found marijuana in his room and suspected that he smoked it regularly. So the positive urine test might not mean much in explaining his recent problems.

Overall, it seemed that there were at least three possibilities for how and why Ronnie had fallen from the rocks and injured himself. He could have become disoriented from the effects of the marijuana, fallen, and knocked himself unconscious from hitting his head on a rock. Alternatively, he could have experienced a seizure, lost consciousness from this (which is common), and then fallen and struck his head. Or he might just been a bit too reckless, miscalculated while climbing over the rocks, and then stumbled and fallen. His grandparents actually thought the last of these was the most likely. Whatever was the cause of his fall, his subsequent unconsciousness likely stemmed from hitting his head.

We can often gauge the timing of injuries by looking at them, and Ronnie's injuries looked to be quite recent. This suggested that he had probably fallen an hour or two before he was found by the hikers. In any event, none of this mattered at the moment for his medical care, so we would just have to ask Ronnie what happened if and when he recovered. He was severely injured, but he was also an extremely lucky boy; many who experience a head injury as bad as Ronnie's was become so comatose that they slow down or even stop their breathing, causing severe further injuries from lack of oxygen to vital organs such as their brain. Although we could not be sure, Ronnie appeared to have escaped that fate.

Thus after Ronnie arrived in the PICU we were still confused about some things, but we still thought that we had the key features of his situation figured out. But, as often happens in the world of the PICU, his situation proceeded to become much more confused; he became far more complicated than just an adolescent with a couple of broken bones and a bonk on the head. So many things were happening at once that it was difficult even for the PICU staff to keep track of everything. In brief, multiple key systems in Ronnie's body began to fail, several of them in life-threatening ways. We had to scramble to manage this organ failure. To complicate things further, it was not clear what caused his deterioration. The best way to narrate the chaos, the "blooming, buzzing confusion" of the next day of Ronnie's life is to tell you the story as one physician would describe it to another—by problem.

Breathing was at the top of Ronnie's immediate problem list. The doctor in the emergency department had placed a breathing tube in Ronnie's airway because he had been concerned that, even though up until then Ronnie had been breathing adequately, it appeared that the child was becoming more comatose, too groggy from his head injury to breathe reliably. And even if Ronnie were breathing enough, comatose patients often are too sleepy to keep their own saliva and mucous out of their airway. Such patients do not cough effectively, causing their breathing passages to get blocked, a life-threatening emergency. For this reason we have a low threshold for intubating comatose patients like Ronnie, even though at that moment there was nothing intrinsically wrong with his lungs themselves. By the time that Ronnie arrived in the PICU several hours later, however, his lungs were no longer normal. We were using increasingly higher pressures on the ventilator and higher concentrations of oxygen in his ventilator to get enough oxygen into Ronnie's bloodstream. We were especially concerned by the speed at which this was happening, since at the rate that he was worsening we would soon reach our maximum settings on the ventilator.

What was going on with Ronnie's lungs? In the last chapter, Robert also developed severe lung failure, but in his case we knew what was going on–acute lung injury from his sepsis syndrome. Things were not so clear with Ronnie. He could indeed have been developing the same thing that had happened to Robert, since the acute lung injury picture can be caused by other things besides the bacteria in Robert's bloodstream that had caused his lung failure. Major trauma, such as Ronnie experienced, is one of those other potential triggers. But there were other possibilities in Ronnie's case, and at least one of these would require us to act quickly to treat it. So time was short; we had to sort through the confusion to figure out what was happening.

Ronnie's bloodstream oxygen situation was deteriorating rapidly and was soon in a terrible state. Usually when this happens an x-ray of the chest shows widespread abnormalities in the lungs which, although they may not tell us exactly what is causing the child's difficulty in getting oxygen into the blood, they at least explain why it is happening. We call the chest x-ray in those situations a "white-out," because all of the places where air should be, and which normally look black on the x-ray, are white because they are filled with fluid that should not be there. Ronnie's chest x-ray, however, did not show a white-out; it surprisingly showed only mild abnormalities. This disparity between Ronnie's blood oxygen content and his x-ray image was so marked that my first impulse when I saw the film was to make sure that the technician had done the correct patient: she had. This suggested that there was little or even nothing wrong with Ronnie's lungs; rather, the problem could be from a blockage of circulation to his lungs so that no blood was flowing there to pick up oxygen. What does that mean?

Our bodies are internal combustion engines. Like a car engine, our bodies take in fuel in the form of food and burn it to produce energy. We constantly need this energy in order to live, and so we continuously need oxygen, because nothing will burn without oxygen. Our lungs take in oxygen with each breath and exhale the byproducts of combustion, which are water and carbon dioxide, each time we breathe out. Our cardiovascular system—our heart pump and the network of blood vessels connected to it—is how our system delivers this vital oxygen to our tissues. So just getting oxygen into our lungs is not enough for us to live; we also require our hearts to pump blood to the lungs to pick up the oxygen, distribute it around the body, and bring back the carbon dioxide to the lungs to be exhaled. So even though Ronnie's lungs might look fine on the x-ray, they were effectively cut off from his body because there was insufficient blood reaching his lungs to get the oxygen. He probably had a blockage of the main vessel going to his lungs, most likely from a blood clot. This is called a pulmonary embolus. Judging from how much trouble we were having getting oxygen into Ronnie's bloodstream, the clot was a big one. What to do?

First, we needed to make sure that Ronnie did indeed have a blockage of blood flow to his lungs. There are several ways to determine this. The safest way is to do a test called a ventilation/perfusion scan. In this test, we inject a radioactive tracer material into the patient's bloodstream and follow its course in the body using a scanner device above the chest; this tells us where the blood flow is going. At the same time, we have the patient breathe in another tracer material, which distributes itself in the airspaces of the lungs; this tells us where the air is going. We then compare these two tracers. The idea is that, if a patient has a pulmonary embolus, a clot blocking the blood flow to the lungs, then there will be areas on the scan that will show the inhaled tracer, but none of the one injected into the bloodstream. We call those lung regions where there is air but no blood areas of "ventilation/perfusion mismatching," and they suggest that something is blocking the blood from flowing there. Scans like this are not overly precise; they are scored as showing a low, intermediate, or high probability of pulmonary embolus. Ronnie's scan came back as "intermediate probability."

This was not very helpful to us, because if he had an embolus in his pulmonary artery, the main vessel leading from his heart to his lungs, we were contemplating using a powerful clot-busting drug to dissolve it. That drug can be dangerous to use, however, so we needed to be sure. The more precise way to determine if a patient has a pulmonary embolus is to inject a substance (radio contrast, or "dye") into the bloodstream and take a rapid series of x-rays (now often done using a CT scanner) to see if anything is blocking movement of the dye through the vessels of the lungs. This test, an angiogram, is riskier to the patient than the ventilation/perfusion scan. Still, Ronnie was critically ill and we needed to know, so we did the test, and it showed a blockage of one of the large vessels leading from his heart to his lungs. Once we knew it was there, we had to decide what to do about it. While we pondered, other problems arose to make Ronnie's situation much more precarious than it already was.

His immediate new problem was that he was bleeding from his broken leg. The femur, the large bone between the hip and the knee, is the largest bone in the body. The very large muscles of the upper leg surround it. When the femur breaks, it often leads to substantial bleeding into those muscles. We were checking Ronnie's blood counts frequently and we knew that he was losing blood, so we suspected that the cause was the broken femur. Because his lung problem was so severe, it would have been to risky for the orthopedic surgeon to take Ronnie to the operating room and fix the femur, which is usually done either by joining the broken ends together with metal plates and screws or by using a metal rod to hold the broken bone ends in alignment with one another until they can heal properly. Since Ronnie could not go to the operating room for one of these definitive fixes, the surgeon aligned the broken ends as best he could by putting Ronnie's leg in traction–stretching his muscles with the simple maneuver of hanging a weight tied to his foot over the end of the bed and pulling the leg straight. Until Ronnie could tolerate the surgery, we would just have to keep giving him blood transfusions and hoping that the bleeding would slow down on its own.

Ronnie's bleeding problem certainly complicated his care. It did, however, resolve the issue of what we could or could not do about his pulmonary embolus. The chief complication from using clot-busting drugs is uncontrollable bleeding. This is because these drugs can bust clots too well; that is, they could dissolve away not only the bad clot in his pulmonary artery, but also other good clots that were helping Ronnie, such as the ones that were stopping the bleeding in his leg. It was already unlikely that we could use these drugs in Ronnie because he appeared to have suffered some bruising on the surface of his brain—we certainly did not want any bleeding there—but the bleeding in his leg settled the issue. We would just have to do the best that we could using the mechanical ventilator and wait for his own body to dissolve the clot in his pulmonary artery as best it could. (We have other ways to handle Ronnie's clot problem now, but his story unfolded before the new technology was available.)

Ronnie soon had other problems besides his lungs. His situation, already complicated, was soon even more complicated. Shortly after he arrived in the PICU, we had placed a tube in his bladder to drain out his urine because comatose patients cannot do that on their own. This tube also allows us to measure how much urine his kidneys were making hour to hour, a measurement that is extremely important when caring for critically ill patients. His nurse noted that Ronnie's urine output had decreased markedly. In addition, his urine had changed color from the normal amber to a pinkish color. Ronnie was going into kidney failure, and the pink urine showed us why. Ronnie was developing complications of a condition termed rhabdomyolosis.

Muscle comprises a large proportion of our body mass. This is particularly so for young, athletic males like Ronnie. One of the principal components of muscle cells is myoglobin, and when many muscle cells are injured, they release large quantities of myoglobin into the bloodstream. The kidneys' main job is to filter waste materials from our blood and eliminate them from our bodies in the urine, so all of the myoglobin goes there for removal. The problem is that even modest concentrations of myoglobin are toxic to the kidneys; large amounts of myoglobin, such as Ronnie had, can cause the kidneys to shut down. Myoglobin is pinkish in color, which was why Ronnie's urine had changed color. It was an ominous sign.

This new development told us that Ronnie had experienced quite a bit of muscle damage, most likely in his legs. That muscle damage was likely caused by one or both of two things: direct injury to the thigh muscles surrounding the broken femur, and indirect damage to the cells from swelling of the muscle. These muscle tissues are separated from one another into bunches by thick bands of fibrous connective tissue, called fascia. These bands have no give or stretch on their own, so if the muscle cells swell, the pressure inside these "compartment" bundles can get too high to allow blood to enter them. When that happens, the muscle cells can die. The orthopedic surgeon used a bedside device to measure the pressure in the compartments of Ronnie's leg and found it too high; if the pressure was not relieved, the muscles cells would soon die.

So, in spite of Ronnie's critically severe lung problem, we had no choice in the matter; we had to take him to the operating room to allow the orthopedic surgeon to relieve the tissue pressure by opening the compartments, decompressing them, with a procedure called a fasciotomy. The anesthesiologist, the physician responsible for Ronnie's lungs and circulation during the surgery, had a tricky time of things just keeping Ronnie alive during the surgery, which the orthopedic surgeon performed as quickly as possible. In spite of this, things were going along reasonably well until the nurse gave Ronnie a dose of a common antibiotic used by surgeons to prevent wounds from becoming infected. This is routine procedure. Nothing, however, seemed to be standard for Ronnie. As if things were not complicated enough for him already, the boy promptly had a severe allergic reaction to the antibiotic–he broke out in hives all over his body, began to have severe wheezing in his lungs, and his blood pressure dropped to a dangerously low level. The anesthesiologist was able to correct all of these problems by promptly giving Ronnie several medicines to reverse the allergic reaction, but unexpected events such as this are particularly dangerous to patients who are already critically ill. What is just a bump in the road for a healthy child can be a killer for a child like Ronnie. But Ronnie's luck held and he made it through the surgery.

As I later described to Ronnie's parents, once Ronnie got back to the PICU, we began several treatments to reduce the damage to his kidneys caused by the myoglobin. Sometimes patients with this problem have their kidneys quit working altogether. When that happens, we need to hook them up to a dialysis machine, a device that does the work of the kidney clearing toxins from the bloodstream. Soon after Ronnie got back to the PICU we asked a kidney expert, a nephrologist, to see him and decide if the boy had enough kidney damage that he needed dialysis already. The nephrologist did not think that Ronnie needed dialysis yet; instead, she suggested that we continue to use the various techniques that we had already started to help flush the myoglobin safely out of Ronnie's system. Even so, we continued to watch the child's kidney function closely, since he might yet need dialysis later.

We next had to turn to the problem of why Ronnie got the blood clot in his lungs in the first place. Even if we could not do anything specific about it, we needed to try to prevent him from getting any new clots there, since another one could easily be fatal for Ronnie. We had already decided that it would be too dangerous to use one of the several drugs that we have to dissolve blood clots because, besides the bleeding in his leg, Ronnie had also suffered some bleeding around his brain. If we gave him one of these drugs to help his lungs, he might well begin to bleed into his brain, causing a severe stroke. It was not worth the risk. There was only one other thing that we could do to help the situation.

Pulmonary emboli, blood clots that appear in the lung's blood vessels and block blood flow, typically are not formed there. Rather, these clots are carried to the lungs from somewhere else. The lungs act as a giant sieve; anything that is in our veins will be carried there and, if it is too large to pass through, trapped in the sieve formed by the lung's meshwork of blood vessels. Pulmonary emboli such as Ronnie had are the result of bits and pieces of clots formed elsewhere breaking loose, being carried downstream in the veins, and then lodging in the sieve of the lungs; the bigger the clot, the bigger the problem, because it is more likely to hang up in a relatively larger, and more important, lung blood vessel. Some of the largest emboli are instantly fatal because they can block all blood flow into the lungs. The source of most of these clots is the large veins in the legs or in the pelvis. We did a few tests that told us that Ronnie had extensive clots in several of these deep veins. They were like ticking time bombs, because if a big one broke loose and went to his lungs it could kill him.

Since clot-dissolving drugs were too dangerous for Ronnie, our only other way to handle the situation was to use a device to catch any

clots that broke loose before they could get to Ronnie's lungs and block
off a big vessel. The device we use for this situation is called an umbrella
filter. It works just like it sounds. Radiologists are usually the physicians
who place them. The radiologist threads the filter, closed up like a rolled
umbrella, through a subsidiary vein until it is positioned in the inferior
vena cava, the large vein that brings blood from the lower part of the
body back to the lungs. Once it is in the correct place, the radiologist
opens the umbrella with its concave surface, analogous to where one
would stand under a real umbrella when holding it over his head, facing
upstream toward where the clots are. The umbrella is made of a material
with millions of tiny holes to let liquid blood flow through, but with
holes small enough such that bits and pieces of clot big enough to cause
problems will be snagged by the filter and prevented from reaching the
lungs. Placing a filter is not a trivial thing, and there are possible complications from them. They also stay in place for the rest of the patient's life,
a key consideration for children. It was not an easy decision. While we
were debating whether Ronnie needed a filter, the boy experienced
another pulmonary embolus. This one thankfully was a smaller one than
his previous one had been, so it did not destabilize him too much. That
second embolus decided things, and he got his filter soon afterwards.

Ronnie had by this time been in the PICU for about twenty-four
hours. He was critically ill. He had been to the operating room once for
major surgery, where he had nearly died from an allergic reaction to a
drug, and to the radiology suite to receive his umbrella filter. His lungs
were in desperate shape, he had experienced a significant injury to his
brain that put him into a coma, and his kidneys were failing. Yet we still
had not been able to speak with his parents, who were traveling in a
remote wilderness area in a time before everyone carried cellular telephones. Ronnie's grandparents had stayed with him in the PICU, but he
really needed his parents, and so did we, because we were finding ourselves forced to do increasingly complicated and potentially dangerous
things to their child as he got sicker and sicker. At last law enforcement
personnel found them out in the backcountry, and they were to arrive
in the PICU the following day.

Up until this point I had been aware of Ronnie's case and had discussed it with my colleagues. My direct involvement, however, had been

only peripheral. That changed the next evening when I took over as the intensivist in charge of the PICU. Different PICUs run things differently depending upon their individual circumstances, but at that time and in that facility each intensivist carried the primary responsibility for running the place for one week at a time. Sometimes that meant that I barely left the PICU for days at a time, and even getting meals and a shower were a problem. At other times things were slow enough that I could catch up on my reading and my paperwork, leave the hospital for half a day or more, and sleep in my own bed without interruption. That is the reality of PICU patient dynamics, and the widely swinging workloads can drive hospital administrators crazy because it is often difficult to plan from day to day how much staff will be needed. Ronnie arrived in the PICU at a time when the PICU census was about average; not too busy, but not too slow either.

When I arrived that evening in the PICU, my colleague who had been in charge for the past week gave me a detailed report of all that had gone one with Ronnie. From her description, it appeared that it would be a long and complicated week in the PICU for both me and for Ronnie. About an hour after I had taken report from my colleague, Ronnie's parents called into the PICU to talk to the doctors. I did the best that I could to explain to his parents everything that was going on with their child, but I told them that I would know a great deal more about the situation when they arrived the next day.

Now that you have been submerged into some of the "blooming, buzzing, confusion" you will probably recognize that feelings of chaos are pretty typical for parents, staff, and even sometimes for the physicians. One aspect of that confusion, at least as it is perceived by parents, is the multitude of doctors involved in caring for complicated children like Ronnie. As I described in Robert's story in the last chapter, this can seem to worsen the chaos. Hand-offs of care, such as occurred when my intensivist colleague turned the case over to me, constitute particular danger points. They can lead to key details being missed, although we do the best that we can to prevent this.

Large university teaching hospitals are institutions that are bustling with many, many doctors in training–interns, residents, and fellows–and it is very difficult for uninitiated outsiders to keep all of these people straight in their minds. All of these young physicians have varying degrees of skills and responsibilities in the PICU. It is the job of the attending intensivist, which in Ronnie's case was me, to supervise and coordinate the activities of all of the members of the PICU team. It is also my responsibility to make sure that you as parents know what is going on with your child, since inevitably you will hear different things from different PICU staff members. However, if your doctor (who may seem overwhelmed with other critical care cases or the many aspects of your child's case) doesn't sit down with you to discuss what is happening, insist on a conference. Amid all the confusion, doctors sometimes need reminding to do just that.

Ronnie's parents arrived in the PICU the next morning. They were exhausted from a long trip. Many parents find themselves feeling extremely tired. If you feel this exhaustion mixed with fear and trepidation, know that such feelings are common. They were in a chaotic mental state. They blamed themselves for having left Ronnie with his grandparents. Like any parent not accustomed to the PICU unit, they were shocked at the sight of their son comatose and hooked up to the PICU life-support machinery. But their unsettled mental and emotional state also stemmed from another cause. Both of Ronnie's parents came from technical, engineering backgrounds. They were used to precise, data-based explanations to physical phenomena, such as what exactly was going on in Ronnie's body. I answered their questions as best I could, but I shared our uncertainty over what was going on inside of their son and what would happen to him. This uncertainty was a particularly difficult thing for them to deal with: "isn't the body like a machine?" his father asked. Over the next day, Ronnie's body was to become less and less a predictable machine and more and more an unpredictable enigma.

Ronnie was fairly stable for a few hours after he got back to the PICU from getting his umbrella filter. Then things began to get complicated again. We had been using various therapies to flush the myoglobin out of his system and protect his kidneys from damage. But in spite of our efforts, his kidney function steadily worsened. The nephrologist decided that it was time to use an artificial kidney machine, a dialysis machine, to do the work of Ronnie's kidneys. I agreed with her assessment of what was needed, even though it meant that I had to place a very large intravenous catheter, one with the diameter of an adult's little finger, in Ronnie's internal jugular vein, the large vein in his neck. Dialysis requires this huge intravenous line to produce sufficient flow of blood through the machine and back to the patient. Placing such a line carries significant risks, particularly for a patient with the lung and bleeding problems that Ronnie had, but fortunately everything went well in his case.

Thus far the list of Ronnie's problems had not included anything with his heart. In fact, it had been doing a great job in spite of the huge stress that Ronnie's body was experiencing. The pulmonary embolus in his lungs had created a particular stress on his heart because the partial blockage of his lung's blood vessels made his heart strain to pump blood against a very high resistance in the system. Ronnie's situation was analogous to someone placing a tight hose clamp around the vessel pipe that came out of his heart and led to his lungs, thereby forcing his heart to pump blood against this constriction. It increased the workload of his heart tremendously, but just the previous day an echocardiogram of Ronnie's heart, a test which tells how well the heart is pumping, showed that his heart was handling the extra work just fine.

This situation began to change around the time that we decided that Ronnie needed dialysis; his heart function began to deteriorate. This is a problem at any time, but it is a particular problem for a patient on dialysis. This is because the dialysis machine demands that we route a significant fraction of the blood in the patient's body to the machine so that it can be treated, cleared of body wastes, and then sent back to the patient. This process can cause wide swings in a patient's blood pressure even if there is nothing wrong with the heart. If the heart is failing, dialysis can cause us huge problems in keeping a patient's blood pressure and entire cardiovascular system on an even keel. We do have a large assortment of drugs that we use to help a failing heart beat more effectively. Robert, in the last chapter, was on some of those drugs. I began Ronnie on one of these medications. But the nephrologist and I had an ominous feeling when we began Ronnie's first dialysis run, a process which takes several hours.

As we anticipated, our ever-more-complicated patient had a rocky time of things during this dialysis treatment. At this point, both Ronnie's parents were at his bedside, and it was particularly difficult for them to watch us manipulating all of the machinery and treatments as his blood pressure and blood oxygen content swung widely back and forth. All of the machinery appeared so precise and sophisticated, yet this belied the imprecision of what we were doing minute to minute. In situations like Ronnie's, seat-of-the-pants intuition and experience are often at least as important as numbers and measurements in managing the patient. In effect, all of the "blooming, buzzing confusion" of the PICU was laid out bare for Ronnie's parents to see. With their technical background, it was an enormous mental struggle for them to watch this happening, but after taking so long to reach their son in the PICU they did not want to leave his bedside.

Ronnie's next dialysis treatment the following day was not as wild as his first one had been. Most important, the dialysis was doing a good job at removing the body wastes from Ronnie's bloodstream. This included the myoglobin that was poisoning his kidneys. But in spite of all of our efforts, Ronnie's kidneys were not healing, even though the myoglobin was mostly eliminated from his system. Worse, we were using higher and higher doses of the drugs that helped his heart to pump more effectively and they were working less and less well. Although it was clear that Ronnie's heart was failing, it was not clear at all why this was happening. The heart experts, the cardiologists, could see and measure this process with their scanning instruments, but none of their tests told them why Ronnie's heart was deteriorating.

By this time Ronnie was being seen daily by a host of organ specialists: he had cardiologists for his heart, nephrologists for his kidneys, neurologists for his brain, pulmonologists for his lungs, orthopedic surgeons for his broken bones, and gastroenterologists for his now failing liver. Each of these experts was accompanied by their own team of doctors-in-training when they came to see Ronnie and his family. As the PICU intensivist, with my own team, my job was to coordinate all of this. All told, nearly thirty physicians were trooping into the PICU each day to see Ronnie. None had really satisfactory answers for Ronnie's parents about what was going on with their son, but I knew addressing their questions was important. Some of them disagreed with one another about what to do. Some of the experts were clear explainers; others spoke to

Ronnie's family using impenetrable medical jargon. If this happens to you, stop them and ask for a clear, understandable explanation. Meanwhile, although his lung function on the ventilator remained fairly stable, the rest of Ronnie's organs continued to dwindle. The overall trend was ominous. As it turned out, it was one of the young trainees, a fellow in gastroenterology, who set us on the path toward figuring out what to do to help Ronnie. Although we may well have arrived at the correct course of action anyway, I have always believed that young physician saved the child's life when he raised the possibility that Ronnie's deterioration could be explained by something we term abdominal compartment syndrome. This particular problem is more widely recognized now in patients like Ronnie than it was at the time when Ronnie was injured, but the concept was understood then.

Abdominal compartment syndrome is analogous to the problem that Ronnie had experienced previously in his leg, and which had needed emergency surgery to fix. The entire abdominal cavity, with all of its organs, can also act as a compartment, one which is encased in relatively inelastic tissues of the surrounding abdominal wall. In some patients these surrounding tissues have a limited ability to tolerate rising pressure inside the compartment. When this pressure gets too high it can interfere with the function of the kidneys, which are just behind the abdominal compartment, and of the heart, which is just above the compartment. It is a difficult diagnosis to make because it is difficult to measure the pressure inside the abdomen. The pressure inside the bladder can serve as a helpful indicator because the bladder experiences much of the intra-abdominal pressure, but abdominal compartment syndrome remains an elusive diagnosis much of the time.

The young gastroenterologist's question set off a debate among the many specialists seeing Ronnie. The stakes in the debate were heightened by the fact that the child's situation was once again deteriorating rapidly. We were supporting his heart and kidneys with all of the technology that we had and it was still not enough. In addition, his lungs, which had been fairly stable, were also worsening. The debate was thus not merely a theoretical one; Ronnie's life might well depend upon the result. Ronnie's parents were experiencing particular psychic strain with all of this because they were well aware that the doctors caring for their son disagreed about what to do. Some of the debates between various physicians were even occurring at Ronnie's bedside for all to hear, and some of the discussions got heated. Although some might see this as an honest way of including Ronnie's parents in the discussion of their child's care, the result was to increase their anxiety immensely. After all, even the doctors did not know what to do!

The gravity of the debate stemmed in part from the fact that the management of abdominal compartment syndrome is not trivial. The only way to relieve the pressure inside the abdomen is for a surgeon to make a long incision down the midline of the patient, from just below the breastbone to just above the pelvic bone. This incision is then covered over with various dressings, but it is left open to allow relief of the pressure. In effect, the abdominal contents–mostly the intestines–spill out from the incision and are protected from the outside world only by dressings. This is not surgery that we undertake lightly. In fact, the surgeon who would have to do the procedure was among the doctors who were not convinced that Ronnie even had abdominal compartment syndrome.

Our discussion about what to do lasted through an afternoon and into the evening. Meanwhile Ronnie continued to worsen. Ultimately all of us, including the surgeon who would actually do it, agreed that the surgery offered Ronnie his best chance to survive and one day walk out of the PICU. Ronnie went down to the operating room later that night. I went with him, both to help the anesthesiologist manage all of Ronnie's problems with his heart, lungs, and kidneys, and because I wanted to know as soon as I could if we had made the correct decision. We had. Soon after the surgeon opened Ronnie's abdominal cavity, the child's heart function began to improve. Within a few hours, his kidney function had improved substantially. I was able to decrease the doses of the drugs that we were using to support Ronnie's heart, and by two days later his kidney function had improved to the point that we no longer needed the dialysis machine.

From that point on Ronnie progressively healed his entire body. It took over a month, but after that night the child never significantly deteriorated again. There were inevitable bumps in the road to recovery–the occasional fever, some transient dips in Ronnie's blood oxygen content and kidney function–but the overall trend was one of steady recovery. The surgeon was able to close the incision in Ronnie's abdomen after four days. Ronnie's lungs continued to heal and he had no more problems with clots in the wrong places. His brain swelling healed on its own. Five weeks after Ronnie had arrived in the PICU, I stopped his sedative medicines, woke him up, and took him off the ventilator.

Ronnie's parents, by now, were getting more used to the PICU, but it was still a strain for them to cope with all of the uncertainty of the place. If, like Ronnie's parents, you are coping with this traumatic circumstance, I remind you to ask questions and discuss your fears and uncertainties with the physician who is captaining the team treating your child. His father, in particular, had a daily battery of questions for my colleagues and I. His questions are a good guide to those you should ask: when will we extubate Ronnie and how will we know that it is time?; how long will it take for him to wake up?; when can he eat?; will he have any more problems with blood clots in his lungs? Will he be able to run and jump like any other child?; will he suffer any longstanding psychological effects from his ordeal? Every reader will suspect what our answers were: we did not know, and only time would tell. That is the reality of PICU medicine.

CRUCIAL ADVICE FOR PARENTS

Coping with confusion and uncertainty is one of the major challenges of having a child in the PICU unit. The more you know, the better you can handle crisis.

Understand that sometimes even the doctors are bewildered and confused.

Prepare in advance for possible child emergencies; confer with your child's doctor on how to do this.

Find out where the nearest PICU unit is and the level of care that it offers.

Keep a copy of your child's medical history at home. If someone else is caring for your child for an extended period, make sure he or she has a copy.

If you hear terms and conditions from medical experts caring for your child that you don't understand, stop them and ask for explanations. Then follow up with some research on your own. Remember, you are your child's best advocate.

Chapter 3

Understanding Supportive
Care's Limits and Advantages

The PICU is filled with amazing technology. You have read how we used this technology to work wonders with the two children in the first chapters. These PICU wonders, however, can make parents, and sometimes even physicians, assume that we have a wonder therapy for nearly every serious ailment that a child might have. This is not so. Sometimes what the PICU provides to children is only an updated version of an ancient and venerated medical tradition–supportive care, the art of watchful waiting at a sick child's bedside while we do our best to relieve the child's pain and discomfort. In those situations we have little control over the outcome; we can only wait and see what will happen, hoping and praying for the best. This chapter tells the story of one such child and the challenge that her mother faced in coming to understand and accept the reality of PICU supportive care.

Tiffany's story is one of a newborn and a breathing problem which we diagnosed to be whooping cough. If you know of anyone who has recently suffered from whooping cough, you know it is not an archaic illness, as many people think, but one that is preventable with a vaccine. Why and how this baby got whooping cough is perhaps the more important story here as compared to her treatment which, as mentioned before, was very much "supportive care," meaning that, simply put, either she would recover—or not.

Tiffany was four weeks old when she first began to cough. It was mild at first; she would cough several times in a row then would seem fine for several hours or more. Over the course of a few days, however, her coughing spells got worse and worse. She would sputter and gasp for air at the end of each spell, and the spells lasted longer and longer. By then she was coughing so much that she was not able to nurse normally. Sometimes she would vomit her feeding at the end of a coughing spell. After several days of these steadily worsening symptoms, Susan, her mother, brought Tiffany to the emergency department of our hospital to find out what was wrong. While they were waiting in the emergency department to see the doctor, the child had her worst coughing spell yet, one which left her purple in the face and gasping for breath. The nurse in the waiting room was very worried about this spell, and called for the doctor to come see Tiffany immediately. He arrived in time to see the spell just ending, but he was so concerned that the child would have more of them and soon be unable to breathe that he brought her immediately back to the examining room.

Once he had Tiffany in the examining room, the doctor gave her extra oxygen to breathe and used a suction tube to suck out the large amount of thick mucous that was clogging the infant's nose and throat and making it extremely hard for her to breathe even between coughing spells. She was dehydrated because she had not nursed very well for most of the day, so the doctor started an intravenous line to give her some needed fluids. Then he sent Tiffany up to the PICU because he was very concerned that her respiratory problems would get so bad that she might ultimately be unable to breathe at all. His concern was well founded.

Tiffany continued to have severe bouts of coughing throughout the afternoon and evening of her first day in the PICU, spells which left her limp and exhausted at the end of each one. Even between these spells, she began to sputter and choke on the progressively larger amounts of phlegm in her nose and throat, mucous which the PICU nurses were constantly sucking from her airway with a plastic tube. Tiffany was too exhausted from all of this coughing to feed well, so we needed to pass a thin plastic tube through her nose and down into her stomach and through which we could give her liquid formula. She began to need more and more oxygen even between her coughing spells. By the morning following her arrival in the PICU, Tiffany was having so much trouble breathing that it appeared we would soon need to place her on a mechanical ventilator. She was just too tired to go on breathing.

Tiffany's lung problem differed in key ways from those of Robert and Ronnie, the children in the previous chapters. Robert's episode of septic shock after his liver transplant made his lungs so stiff that they could not do their job of getting oxygen into his blood stream. Ronnie had a pulmonary embolus, a blockage in the blood flowing to the lungs from the heart. Tiffany's breathing difficulty was of a different sort; her problem was blockage of her airway such that air could not even get into her lungs. Her bronchi, the small breathing tubes that carry air from the mouth and nose down into the lungs, were clogged with debris. She was so small and had been struggling so long to cough all of that material out of her lungs that it appeared likely that she would soon just wear out and quit breathing altogether from sheer exhaustion. What was wrong with Tiffany? Why was she coughing so much, and where was all of the mucous coming from?

By the morning after Tiffany's admission to the PICU, tests showed us for certain what her problem was, although her very characteristic symptoms had made us highly suspicious of the cause even before we knew for sure. The doctor in the emergency department had sent some of Tiffany's infected respiratory secretions to the laboratory for testing, and the results showed that Tiffany had whooping cough, also called pertussis after *Bordetella pertussis*, the scientific name for the bacteria that usually causes the illness.

The infection affects children in several ways. Our respiratory tract normally produces mucous every day. This is one of the key ways that we protect our lungs from all of the particles in the air, such as dirt, pollen, and dust. When we breathe these particles in, they are trapped by the mucous in our airways, and we then cough the material out, which is why our phlegm looks dark after we have been in a dusty environment. The whooping cough bacteria increase the amount of mucous in the infected child's airway. In addition to that, the bacteria interfere with how the lungs normally get mucous up from the small airways to cough it out. The result is that a child with whooping couch is nearly drowning and gasping for air between coughs; this gasp at the end of a coughing spell is the "whoop" of whooping cough. Most persons mistakenly think of whooping cough as a relic from their grandparents' era. This is not true; we see several cases in the PICU every year.

But how did Tiffany get whooping cough? She was a young infant who had barely been out of her house. She had not gone any place where she might have been exposed to sick people. The answer is that she caught it from someone who was infected with the germ and who brought it to her. The local public health department later did an investigation, as is routine for communicable diseases like whooping cough, and determined that she had caught it from a six-year-old neighbor boy who had come to her house to play with Tiffany's brother. The boy had himself been coughing for weeks, but older children generally do not have the severe symptoms from whooping cough that infants do, so his parents never took him to the doctor. And why did this boy get the infection? His parents did not believe in vaccinations, and so he had never received any.

We have a vaccine to prevent whooping cough. This vaccine, however, has caused some controversy. This is because the form of the vaccine that doctors used for many years, although effective, also caused a substantial amount of discomfort to the children who received it, mostly in the form of pain at the injection site and fever. Very few children—perhaps one or two each year in the entire county—showed more severe reactions. Some of these children may have suffered brain damage, although validated research on the question has never shown any clear link between the whooping cough vaccine and permanent damage to children. Still, the issue generated a great deal of attention in the press, and concern over the possibility of injury caused some parents to withhold the vaccine from their children.

These days, however, we have a new whooping cough vaccine that does not cause the reactions that the old one did, particularly the high fever. Yet in spite of this high-tech breakthrough, some parents still refuse to vaccinate their children. I have talked to many such parents and have listened to their reasons for not trusting the vaccines. Although I am sympathetic to their viewpoint, I think that they are wrong. I also think that they are putting both their children and innocent children like Tiffany at risk for serious or life-threatening infection. As you might expect, Tiffany's mother had stronger opinions than mine on the matter of vaccinations. She was more than unsympathetic to the anti-vaccination viewpoint; she was scornful of its adherents, even angry at them. She told me that she would like all such parents who refuse whooping cough vaccine for their children to see a video of Tiffany, emaciated from lack of food, exhausted from coughing, and nearly drowning in mucous as she gasped to breathe. Before the vaccine became available in the 1950s, there were hundreds of thousands of cases of whooping cough each year in the United States, and some of these children died or suffered permanent damage from the infection. After the first vaccine was introduced, the number of cases plummeted, but there are still nearly ten thousand cases each year in the United States, and the number is rising. Thirteen children died from whooping cough in 2003. One reason for the rise in cases is incomplete vaccination among small children, but the other reason is that our present vaccine does not give life-long protection from the infection, so adolescents and adults can get whooping cough when the immunity conferred by their initial, childhood vaccinations has worn off. Many, even most cases occurring today are seen in that population of older persons. Public health researchers are presently debating over what to do about this, and many have called for periodic booster vaccinations for adolescents and adults. But Tiffany did not catch whooping cough from a previously vaccinated older person whose immunity had waned; she got it from a deliberately unvaccinated child.

Tiffany's story shows you something else, something that points out an important challenge for those of us who work in the PICU. Children, especially infants, are difficult little creatures to evaluate and assess their degree of discomfort. They fuss and cry, of course, but pound-for-pound, young children willingly suffer far more pain and anguish than an adult will without complaint. This is true for more than pain; it is particularly so with breathing problems. Therefore physicians and nurses who work in the PICU must be able to anticipate when a child in respiratory distress is getting into dangerous breathing trouble, and they must make the decision using only minimal data. Objective measurements, such as how fast the child is breathing and how much oxygen is needed, are useful and can help us make this decision, but ultimately technology is of little help; it takes experience and fine judgment. In fact, the best indicator of serious respiratory deterioration in a child is simply when an experienced observer, using his or her own sixth sense for these things, judges that a child's breathing is failing.

Part of the difficulty in making this judgment is that infants and small children with respiratory distress, whether the cause is asthma, pneumonia, or some other problem, typically do not worsen in a steady progression; rather, they tend to hold their own for a considerable time, then collapse all at once. Children often compensate in their breathing in such a way that, even though their lung problem is steadily worsening, they appear superficially unchanged until they suddenly deteriorate in life-threatening ways. All of us aim to anticipate this sudden deterioration and head off the potential catastrophe yet do so without overreacting and placing every child on a ventilator who might conceivably need one. In practice, this distinction represents a very fine line to walk. Doing it well is one of the key aspects of the art of pediatric critical care practice.

In Tiffany's case, it was obvious by the afternoon of her second day in the PICU that she was progressively becoming too exhausted from coughing to breathe effectively much longer. She was limp and listless much of the time. Her cry was weak. She stopped feeding altogether. Her eyes were puffy and swollen, their whites bloodshot from all of her coughing. Like Robert and Ronnie in the previous chapters, it was clear that she needed our most common PICU high-tech device–the mechanical ventilator machine. Putting her on a ventilator would allow us to sedate her with medications so that she could rest and recuperate while the machine did all of the work of breathing for her. There was another important reason to intubate Tiffany: we could then also use the breathing tube to get the mucous out of her lungs that she could not cough up herself.

If your baby or young child needs to be intubated (put on a mechanical ventilator), you should know that this is not without risk; in fact, the risks are significant, and you should have your child's doctor talk to you about them and about the steps of the procedure. The key point is that, for Tiffany, it was a greater risk for her to be off the ventilator than on it. Some intubations are riskier than others. Tiffany's situation— that of a small infant with mucous-clogged airway—made her intubation a relatively higher-risk, complicated procedure.

As I did with Robert, the child in the previous chapter, my first step in placing Tiffany on a ventilator was to use a mask to give her pure, one hundred percent oxygen to breathe for a few minutes. This filled her lungs with a reserve supply of oxygen in case any problems are encountered. (For comparison, the air we breathe is only twenty-one percent oxygen; the balance is mostly nitrogen.) Once her lungs were full of oxygen, I then gave her an anesthetic drug through her intravenous line.

When the drug took effect in Tiffany's system, she instantly stopped breathing. This often happens in small infants, but it meant that I had to breathe for her using a mask. I then placed the mask over her mouth and nose, which attached to a bag filled with oxygen. I then squeezed the bag to deliver each breath into her lungs. At that point Tiffany was asleep from the anesthetic and I could easily ventilate her lungs with the bag and mask. As I had done with Robert, I next gave Tiffany a drug to relax her muscles and waited the minute or so that it takes the relaxing drug to act, meanwhile continuing to breathe for her with the bag and mask.

Suddenly, just about the time that the relaxing drug was taking effect, all of the monitors went awry as Tiffany's blood oxygen content nose-dived and her heart rate slowed to a dangerous level. At the same moment, I was suddenly unable to ventilate her with the bag and mask, meaning that her chest was not moving up and down as it should with each squeeze. Something was blocking the air from getting into her lungs and no oxygen was reaching her bloodstream. Her heart was already suffering from this lack of oxygen, and it showed this by slowing down to an abnormal degree. If this situation persisted, Tiffany would die within a few minutes.

Since Tiffany was in a relaxed state from the medication that I had given her, it was relatively easy for me to insert the laryngoscope into her mouth and use the light on the end to get a good view of her upper airway. The problem was obvious immediately; there was a large chunk of mucous blocking the opening to her windpipe, the trachea. Tiffany's nurse handed me a suction device to clear the obstruction and I was then able to pass the tube into her trachea, connect it to the oxygen bag, and give Tiffany a few breaths of pure oxygen. Tiffany's blood oxygen content and heart rate bounced back to normal within a few seconds and the alarms on the monitors stopped clanging.

Even after this crisis had passed, I still was having some difficulty getting Tiffany's chest to move up and down when I squeezed the bag, and I suspected that it was because of the thick mucous deep in her breathing passages. This proved to be exactly the case. The debris from the whooping cough had been building up in her lungs for days, blocking her ability to breathe. There was so much of it that the nurse needed to make several passes down the breathing tube with the suction catheter to clear Tiffany's airway. When we were finished, Tiffany's chest moved much better with each breath from the ventilator. Our experience has taught us that this improvement was only temporary, because infants with whooping cough continue to produce large amounts of mucous. Tiffany, like most infants in this situation, would need to have her breathing tube suctioned at least every few hours to keep it clear.

Parents need to know that there is really no such thing as a routine intubation for an infant or child critically ill with severe breathing or airway problems. We must be ready for all sorts of potential disasters. For example, trouble may start right from the beginning if the child experiences a strange reaction to the anesthetic or relaxing medications. In some cases, the child may vomit stomach contents and get some of this material down into the airway or lungs, although we take various precautions to reduce the chances of this happening.

Once I had secured Tiffany's airway with the endotracheal tube, I needed to secure lines placed in her blood vessels to monitor how her blood oxygen and heart function were doing. She also needed a small tube placed through her nostril down into her stomach to prevent her from becoming bloated with air, and through which we could feed her. I inserted these devices once Tiffany was stable on the ventilator.

Using drugs on children as small as Tiffany takes precise judgment and an understanding of how infants and children handle pain. I needed to relieve her discomfort of being on a ventilator and having all of those tubes and lines, as well as reduce any anxiety caused by the whole experience. Although she was an infant, we presumed that she would experience the discomfort and anxiety from what we were doing to her in much the same way that an older person would. Both the children in the earlier chapters were in fairly deep comas when they went on the ventilators, so their need for sedatives was modest. In contrast, Tiffany was wide awake when I prepared to intubate her. I used a general anesthetic drug for the intubation procedure itself, but that medication wears off quickly. Once it does, we typically use a combination of a narcotic pain killer and one of several anti-anxiety drugs similar to Valium to relieve pain and distress.

Once Tiffany was intubated and on the ventilator I gave her continuing doses of medications to keep her comfortable. In truth, for several days she hardly needed them because, once on the ventilator, she promptly did what many infants in her situation do—she let the machine do all of her breathing. The best evidence of how hard Tiffany's struggle over the past week had been for her was her weight; when I intubated her, she barely weighed more than she had at birth, having spent all of her precious calories on coughing, rather than on growing.

Pediatric intensive care practice has made great strides in the last decades regarding how we treat pain and anxiety in infants and children. At one time, physicians had an irrational fear of addicting children to pain killers and were reluctant to use them. Incredible as it seems to us now, some physicians even questioned whether or not small children even experienced pain in the same way that adults do. Years ago children like Tiffany were simply restrained in their bed to prevent them from pulling out their lines and tubes and were not given any sedatives at all. We now know that infants and young children do experience pain in similar ways to older persons, and that addiction and future drug problems do not occur when these medicines are used in the PICU situation. Doctors today believe it is wrong to deny children the comfort that these medications can give, and which any adult in that situation would demand.

If you as parents are uneasy with the thought of your baby or young child being medicated, know this: providing adequate pain medicine has deeper implications than just practicing humane medicine; stress and pain are hard on the body. In fact, research has shown that managing pain well makes a child heal faster. This is because pain and anxiety cause the release of stress hormones, a reflex which constitutes our body's "fight or flight" response. These hormones allow our bodies to achieve great feats of endurance, but they do so by cannibalizing our internal organs for fuel and nutrients. High levels of stress hormones in a critically ill child's system block tissue healing. These are scientific issues regarding pain relief. My own goal when I sedate a critically ill child is for that child to have no memory of who I am when he or she awakens. If that happens, then I know that the child will likely have minimal recollection of everything else that happened while under sedation.

Tiffany was quite stable once she was on the ventilator with all of her life support lines in place. Her need for what the ventilator could do, the pressure that the machine needed to use in order to breathe for her, was in the modest range for infants her size. She continued to have very large amounts of mucous in her lungs, so she also needed the breathing tube to allow us to clean the material from her airway. But could we do any more than that? Was there any specific treatment, such as antibiotics, that could cure Tiffany's illness? After all, whooping cough is a bacterial infection and we have many powerful antibiotics to treat bacterial infections.

The answer to this question, unfortunately, is no. Once whooping cough has become established in a child, once the characteristic coughing spells have begun, no antibiotic will help the symptoms. We do give children like Tiffany an antibiotic (either erythromycin or a drug related to it), but this only prevents the child from infecting others by removing the bacteria from the mucous secretions. Even though one would intuitively expect that clearing the bacteria from the child's system would help the situation, it does not appreciably do so. We also give erythromycin to any close contacts of a child with whooping cough, such as family members, since research has found that they are often carrying the bacteria in their throats whether or not they have symptoms of any illness. We do this to block the chain of infection. But it is a distressing fact that once the coughing phase of the illness has started, the disease runs its course no matter what we do. This stresses the importance of getting your children all the vaccinations that your doctor recommends.

Our inability to do anything directly to cure Tiffany points out a frustrating fact for doctors and a challenge for her mother. Tiffany's dilemma teaches us about the limits of what high-tech, PICU care can and cannot do. For Robert, the child with liver failure, we had amazing and specific treatments for what was wrong with him. I had no such wonderful treatments to offer Tiffany. All that I could do was to supply her with a ventilator to breathe, use the endotracheal tube to suck the mucous from her lungs, and use the tube through her nose into her stomach to feed her. We would need to do these things for as long as it took for the whooping cough to run its course. Tiffany's story teaches us that for many PICU patients, all of our high-tech care is what we call only supportive; that is, we use it both to support the child's vital organ function as best we can and to relieve pain and discomfort. But we can do nothing to cure the child; he or she will either recover or not. Tiffany was this sort of patient. This reality is a huge challenge for parents who suddenly and unexpectedly find themselves in the position of Tiffany's mother to grasp this truth and accept it.

What we were doing for Tiffany looked, at first glance, to be modern and high-tech. In fact, we were doing the things that are as old as the practice of medicine itself. After all, comforting the sick, giving pain-relieving remedies when needed, feeding the patient properly, and ultimately waiting out the course of an illness at a patient's bedside with a concerned family are traditions of care that date back to the time of Hippocrates. For children like Tiffany, PICU care consists of little more than a modern manifestation of this ancient tradition. Our tools have become highly sophisticated, but the bedside drama of watching a sick patient wrestle with illness or injury has, for many children, changed little over the millennia. Tiffany teaches us a key truth about PICU: nowhere is humanistic medical practice more important than in the intensive care unit, medicine's most technologically sophisticated setting. The hissing of ventilators and the beeping of monitors sometimes tend to obscure that reality.

Some parents are surprised by this state of affairs. They see only the limitations of supportive care, and are frustrated by those limitations. They look around them in the PICU and see the full array of high-tech machinery available and are astonished that we do not have a specific treatment for nearly anything. Parents are sometimes more than frustrated by this truth; some are even angry about it. I have often been asked by these parents, "Doctor, can't you *do* anything to help?"

And herein lay the trust issue. If the trust in the PICU is lacking, then a child's family is more likely to assume that the doctors do not know enough. After all, just because their child's doctor does not know of any specific treatments that might help does not mean that there *are* no treatments available. Sometimes families are right; doctors don't know everything. My own experience has been that, if I have been speaking with a child's family regularly to explain what is going on and to answer their questions then this issue rarely arises. However, if a family really has concerns about my management of their child's illness, I always suggest that we consult other physicians to get other opinions. In fact, I have found that my willingness to suggest this to a family often restores whatever trust has been lost between the PICU team and the family.

Even though some parents find the very notion of "only" supportive care frustrating, many other parents do not. It has been my experience that many families, perhaps even the majority of them, paradoxically find a form of comfort in our lack of a specific cure for their child. I believe that this is because the ancient practice of waiting patiently at the bedside until recovery either happens or does not happen restores a measure of control to parents, who often feel quite powerless in the PICU environment. Supportive care and watchful waiting leave substantial room for non-medical measures such as hope, love, and prayer to work their wonders. These are best provided by a child's family, not by the doctors and nurses. The situations of children like Tiffany seem to carry with them a real feeling of partnership between families and PICU staff because each has their own sphere of expertise, their own job to do. Each has their own variety of supportive care to give to the child.

It was nearly a week before the amount of mucus in Tiffany's lungs had subsided to the point where we could begin weaning her from the ventilator. During this time we had been feeding her high-potency infant formula and she had managed to regain a good measure of her lost weight. Although she was still on the ventilator, she was doing more and more of the breathing herself as her strength returned. This is possible because we can turn down the ventilators, gradually allowing the child to breathe on his or her own through the endotracheal tube. Tiffany was making good progress in this process of weaning from the ventilator.

There are some objective measurements that help us decide when it is time to take a child off the machine, particularly an infant, but ultimately experience and judgment rule. My colleagues and I agreed that after some ten days on the machine, it was time to take the plunge and see if Tiffany could breathe without the ventilator.

As I did with Robert and Ronnie, whose experiences I highlighted in the previous chapters, I began the process of weaning Tiffany from the ventilator by reducing her doses of the sedative medications. We need to get these drugs out of a child's system because virtually all of them interfere with normal, spontaneous breathing. They do this by dulling the brain's response to the state of either having not enough oxygen or too much carbon dioxide in the bloodstream. Normally either of these things, particularly the latter, stimulates us to breathe. Sedative drugs blunt this normal reflex, although it is true that children who have been on these medications for days or weeks develop some tolerance to this effect on their spontaneous breathing. The degree of this tolerance is unpredictable from child to child, and the drugs must have their doses reduced gradually. One does not know in advance how much of a problem this will be for the ventilator weaning process of a particular child. My first step in getting Tiffany off the ventilator was to discover this by reducing the doses of the drugs to the point where they did not appear to be interfering with her breathing, but which did not produce any acute withdrawal symptoms. This took me about two days to accomplish.

By the morning of the second day it was time to try to extubate Tiffany. Her mother, Susan, of course, was pleased by her child's progress. She was excited to get her child back in her arms. But she was also nervous, as many parents are when their small children are ready to be extubated. Sometimes parents even plead with me *not* to extubate their children, or to at least delay the procedure. This is because, compared with what Tiffany had gone through before being intubated, her time on the ventilator had been relatively tranquil. Susan, like many parents, had become accustomed to all of the PICU technology and even found comfort in the beeping and hissing of the machinery. Unlike Robert and Ronnie in the previous chapters, Tiffany never experienced a nerve-wracking time of frequent, life-threatening crises in her situation. The condition of her lungs never remotely approached the severity of Robert's lung disease when he was on the oscillator or of Ronnie when he was throwing blood clots to his lungs.

So, although Susan knew it was time to try to take Tiffany off the machine, she was nervous about changing her daughter's now stable condition. In truth, I was a little nervous myself. Sometimes children, particularly infants, fail to make it off the ventilator even when everything seems right for us to extubate them. Still, we needed to try because, even though Tiffany and her mother had gotten used to the ventilator, this technology is not entirely innocent; remaining on a ventilator for several days carries risks of its own, risks which increase the longer that the child is on the machine

Much like intubation, extubation is a multi-step process, one that can pose many problems. When the time comes, doctors do several things to prepare a child like Tiffany for extubation and to maximize the chances of staying off the machine. First, we reduce the doses of the sedatives as I had done during the previous day. This can be a tricky business because, as I noted, we cannot stop the sedatives completely. To do that would be cruel. It would also put the child at risk for developing severe agitation from the abrupt withdrawal of the drugs. When we are getting close to the time of extubation, we stop feeding the child several hours before so that her stomach is empty (we do not want a newly extubated child to vomit and get food down into their lungs). This event, termed aspiration of stomach contents or aspiration pneumonia, is a serious complication that can occur whenever a child's airway is manipulated.

Another problem that can occur after extubation is dangerous narrowing of the airway because of swelling of the tissues there. A child on a ventilator has spent days or even weeks with a plastic endotracheal tube passing between her vocal cords and down into her trachea. The tube inevitably bumps and bangs against the sensitive tissues in the airway whenever the child moves, irritating these tissues to some degree and causing them to swell. When we take out the endotracheal tube, this swelling can be so severe that it closes off the airway where the tube had been. If that happens, we are forced to put the breathing tube back in so the child can breathe, even though we recognize that doing so only puts us back in the same situation; the tube will again irritate the airway, and that irritation can make the swelling even worse. Still, at times like that we have no choice but to intubate the child again; the smaller the child, the smaller the airway and the bigger the potential problem with airway swelling.

When this scenario of severe airway swelling happens, we call it "post-extubation croup," because its symptoms—a raspy, barky cough and difficulty getting air into the lungs—resemble a severe case of the ordinary viral croup that many children experience at one time or another when a respiratory virus causes swelling around their vocal cords. There are a few things that we can do to reduce the chances of this occurring. Drugs, given in advance of extubation, can help reduce the tissue swelling and thus reduce the chances of a child getting post-extubation croup. I gave Tiffany a dose of such a drug called dexamethasone.

Once I had finished all of this, it was time to extubate Tiffany. I gave her a few big extra breaths with my hand ventilation bag and then pulled out the endotracheal tube. She coughed and sputtered a few times and then held her breath for twenty seconds or so, causing both me and Susan several anxious moments. Then she began to breathe normally, if a bit faster than is normal for an infant her age. Even though Tiffany was not on the ventilator, she still needed oxygen, which we gave her through soft plastic prongs that fit into her nose. I did not plan to start feeding her yet because I needed to see how things would go, and her stomach had to remain empty until I was sure that I was not going to need to put the breathing tube back.

As the next few hours progressed, things did not go well for Tiffany. It was soon obvious that she was developing post-extubation croup. First came the barky cough, then, as her airway got smaller and smaller, Tiffany worked harder and harder to breathe. The effect was as if the child were breathing through a straw—an increasingly narrow straw. Her little chest wall moved the wrong way with each breath, back toward her spine, because she was sucking harder and harder to draw air into her lungs. Sometimes a breathing treatment with an inhaled medicine improves post-extubation croup dramatically. I tried this several times, but it did not help her much; after a few hours of worsening struggle it was clear I was going to have to intubate Tiffany again. The child simply could not breathe on her own.

Susan had been holding up under the strain of Tiffany's prolonged, several week illness quite nicely. She was eating and sleeping reasonably well, and had good support from a circle of devoted friends, most of whom were mothers of small children themselves. These friends visited the PICU frequently, and one of them was there the morning that I extubated Tiffany. But Tiffany's most recent struggle after her extubation was too much for Susan, and she became extremely upset. She alternated between fury at the unfairness of the whole situation and focused anger at the family of the child who had given Tiffany whooping cough.

Susan was also more than a little angry at me, a turn of events which often happens in PICU situations like this. Even though I had explained to Susan that Tiffany might not make it off the ventilator on her first try, and justified my reasons for trying to extubate her that morning, my explanations were abstract, in a sense, because Susan had assumed that her daughter would do fine. This was a hopeful and appropriate assumption, but it was wrong. Now Susan was angry and I was the obvious target.

It is quite normal for parents to feel rage and hopelessness at the injustice of a situation such as this one, and in turn take it out on the doctors and nurses. The PICU can be extraordinarily stressful for parents, and I often think they are more calm, composed, and understanding than they should be considering the circumstances. From a doctor's viewpoint, I let them vent their frustration as long as they need to, as long as it does not interfere with the care of their child or the other children in the PICU. This does happen sometimes. I have worked in PICUs that are quite cramped, and have encountered situations when altercations within and between families and staff have caused problems. That was not the case with Susan, whose experience in the PICU stresses the importance of having close friends and family members who can offer comfort and support at such an emotional time. It is very, very hard to go through this alone.

Susan cried for a time then apologized to me, as most parents do after they vent their anger; after all, she only wanted Tiffany to get better, and this seemed like such a setback. She was also so accustomed to the PICU now that, unlike the first time, Susan wanted to stay and watch while I intubated Tiffany. This time Tiffany was much better overall and the procedure went smoothly. However, I could see when I looked with my laryngoscope that her airway tissues were swollen and red, so the diagnosis of post-extubation croup was the correct one. But at least all of the mucous from the whooping cough had gone. She was sufficiently improved that I could use an endotracheal tube that was a bit smaller than the previous one. This helped the swelling from getting worse because the smaller tube would be less irritating. I also gave Tiffany several more doses of dexamethasone to reduce the swelling.

By the next day her airway swelling was much improved, and it was time to try to take her off the ventilator once more. If Susan had been nervous before the last extubation, she was *really* nervous now. Thankfully, this time all went well. When I pulled out the breathing tube Tiffany had only a few modest retractions of her chest wall, nothing as severe as before. Her situation was still tenuous for the next twelve hours or so, and we had to give her several breathing treatments for croup to reduce the swelling. But little by little, Tiffany breathed easier. By the next morning she was breathing fine.

Although the huge quantities of mucous in her lungs had resolved,

Tiffany still coughed a great deal. It was now a dry cough, and it still tended to come in bursts. This is very common after whooping cough. Children may even have repeated bouts of severe coughing months later if they contract another respiratory infection, such as a simple cold virus. Whooping cough is a severe condition, not to be underestimated or dismissed as a "childhood illness." In Tiffany's case, even though her continuing cough was not as bad as it had been before she first went on the ventilator, it was still too severe to allow her to eat. The cough also left her too exhausted to even try to eat, so she would still need her feedings to go through the tube in her nose down into her stomach.

Supportive care is what we were still providing for Tiffany. There was nothing specific that we could do to reduce the frequency or intensity of her coughing spells. Tiffany was still in a lot of trouble. Days went by in which she did not gain any weight at all because, in spite of the calorie-rich formula that we were giving her through her feeding tube, her coughing spells used up all of her energy. After about a week of this she at last began to gain weight steadily. Gradually her coughing spells got shorter and less frequent. We began to feed at least a portion of her daily formula using a bottle, and her ability to suck on the bottle got stronger and stronger. Three weeks after her extubation she was taking all of her feedings by bottle so we removed the plastic tube from her nose. Finally, after six weeks in the hospital, Tiffany was well enough to go home with her mother.

Most children heal well. This fact is what makes much of what we do in the PICU possible. It is astonishing how, given the chance, a great number of children can recover from an illness or injury that would kill an adult. Tiffany's story shows how durable infants and children are if we provide them with needed life support measures, fluids and nutrition, and then simply wait for them to heal. For children like Tiffany, the PICU represents a modern, high-tech twist on an ancient medical practice. I hope for those parents who are learning of its functions, this is a comforting and rewarding fact.

CRUCIAL ADVICE FOR PARENTS

Trust your instincts with babies and small children. If, for instance, you think your infant is working too hard to breathe, don't wait— bring the baby immediately to the doctor.

Be aware of the physical condition of friends and acquaintances and who you introduce your baby to in those first important weeks of life. Keep away anyone with signs of a cough or cold. The best way to stop the spread of infection is to wash your hands often with soap and water.

Vaccinate your children and don't forget about booster shots. While it may be slightly uncomfortable for the child, the benefits outweigh the disadvantages. By refusing vaccinations for your child, you are putting him or her at risk for a life-threatening infection. As Tiffany's story showed, vaccinations also protect children other than your own.

Understand that although your child is an infant, he or she still suffers pain and will most likely benefit from pain medication. Managing pain makes a child heal faster. If you think that your child is in excessive pain, discuss it with your doctor.

Learn about the disease your child is faced with. In this case, realize whooping cough cannot be treated with antibiotics.

Recognize the limits of PICU hi-tech care. Sometimes, it's just "supportive care" we offer; sometimes it just comes down to if the child will either recover or not—a hard fact that parents have to understand and accept.

Understand and manage your anger and frustration. Know it is normal to be annoyed when doctors' predictions don't turn out right. Sometimes waiting a problem out is the only choice.

If you have concerns about a physician managing your child's illness, don't be afraid about consulting with other physicians to get a second opinion.

Prayer, hope and love are important PICU therapies too, and these are best provided by the family.

Don't underestimate the support of friends and family.

Chapter 4

Doing the Right Thing

The PICU is a place of life and death decisions, and life and death decisions demand an ethical sense. This is why the PICU is a focal point for some of the most difficult moments in medical practice. This fact highlights one of the chief ironies of our health care system: humanistic and ethical issues—questions that are as old as medical practice itself—are especially prominent in medicine's most modern and technologically advanced setting. These ethical questions often have no clear answers. This can lead to disagreements among members of the PICU staff, between PICU staff and families, and among family members. They often arise from deeply-held opinions, and they can be bitterly divisive. For those of us who work in the PICU, we must understand and mediate the inevitable controversies that surround ethical questions. To do that we need more than just our own deeply held opinions; we also require a guiding frame of reference, one that comes from having a practical grasp of medical ethics.

This chapter introduces you to how families and staff in the PICU struggle to apply ethical principles in real-life situations; in this case, how one family used these principles to make difficult choices for their son, Cody, who was diagnosed with a severe genetic defect called spinal muscular atrophy. His story not only delves into medical ethics but, most importantly, deals with experienced intensivists and their occasional encounters with black and white distinctions between right and wrong. Life, as experienced in the PICU, is far more complicated than Hollywood

script writers depict it. This is not a bad thing, because it is through grap-
pling with real-life ethical and moral issues, with all their complexities and
ambiguities, that we can truly become more human.

If you are in such a distressing situation where you must make a
life and death decision for your child, acquaint yourself with the many
gray areas of quality-of-life issues. Get in touch with your personally-
held beliefs on the subject. What would you do for your child if faced
with a life-threatening situation? Would your spouse agree? Be aware
that, as noted previously, such predicaments will tear some families apart.
It is important to stress here the need for communication among family members.

Cody was two months old when his parents brought him to the
emergency department of our hospital one Saturday morning. They
noticed their child had been having difficulty breathing the past few
days—his breaths seemed to be labored, too rapid, and shallow. He
seemed weak and listless to them and had not been feeding normally.
That morning Cody's fever and cough were bad enough that his parents
took him to the ER instead of waiting for their scheduled doctor's
appointment. The physician in the emergency room noted that Cody
indeed had a fever, was breathing too fast, and had a reduced amount of
oxygen in his bloodstream. Cody's chest x-ray showed what the problem was: he had pneumonia. The physician gave Cody oxygen, started
an intravenous line to give him fluids and antibiotics, and called me to
ask for a bed in the PICU because it appeared to him that Cody was
quite weak and might need intensive care to help him breathe.

After Cody arrived in the PICU it did not take long for us to discover the fundamental problem: he was extremely weak. Cody's parents
told me that over the past few weeks the strength of his suck on his bottle had gotten progressively weaker, so that he was taking longer and
longer to finish the same amount of formula. They were afraid that he had
lost some weight. They also had noted that he seemed to move less and
less in his crib. When I examined Cody I easily heard through my stethoscope the characteristic bubbling sounds of his pneumonia. I expected to
find that. But what was particularly striking to me was how weak Cody
was. A normal newborn can lift his head and move it from side to side
when lying on his stomach and Cody's parents told me that the child

could do this when he was born. Now, however, Cody was completely unable to lift his face off the mattress when lying on his stomach.

When I examined Cody further, I found other disturbing signs. His deep tendon reflexes—the involuntary twitches of the limbs one elicits by tapping the knees or elbows with a rubber hammer to make them jerk—were gone. Cody's most striking abnormality was obvious when I opened his mouth—the surface of his tongue was rippling back and forth in wormlike movements called fasiculations. These movements are characteristic of patients with Cody's type of problem. Taken together, all of these things showed that the nerves connecting Cody's muscles to his brain were dying off. And without a supply of nerves, the muscles themselves also die and disappear, a process termed atrophy. His neurological problem had also caused his pneumonia, because his progressive weakness as his muscles atrophied made it harder and harder both for him to cough up the mucous normally produced by his lungs, and to keep his feedings from getting down into his airway when he swallowed. Such weakness leads to a form of pneumonia called aspiration pneumonia, and that is what had landed Cody in the PICU.

Cody had a condition called spinal muscular atrophy. The disease comes in several varieties. Cody's form, also called Werdnig-Hoffman disease, is the most severe of these. It has very characteristic physical findings, which are usually confirmed with a blood test. The fundamental problem in this disease is that the motor neurons—the nerves that supply the muscles and tells them when to contract—progressively die off.

Spinal muscular atrophy is a malfunction in how the nervous system develops. When we are embryos, barely a month after conception, we have many more of the kind of precursor cells (that later become motor neurons) than we need. As our nervous systems develop and mature the extra and unneeded neurons, amounting to about half of the precursor cells, die off. This process, called apoptosis or programmed cell death, continues until we have just the right amount for our nervous systems. This delicate and complicated process is regulated by genes that are just now being studied and understood.

Children with spinal muscular atrophy have a defect in how this finely balanced system is controlled. Instead of stopping at just the right time, the process of motor neuron death continues unchecked until virtually all of them are gone. A malfunction in the gene that normally tells the process to stop is the cause. The speed at which this progressive motor neuronal death occurs varies from child to child. Although brain researchers are trying to devise therapies to slow down or even stop the process, they are working against all odds with Cody's form of the disease where the loss of motor neurons is rapidly relentless, ultimately leaving the child unable to move, cough, or even breathe. When that happens, we can keep such a child alive, but we can do nothing about the underlying neurological problem.

With children like Cody, we now have the technology to treat their pneumonia and respiratory failure and to feed them when they become too weak to eat. We can perform a tracheostomy, a procedure in which a surgeon makes a cut in the trachea (windpipe) just below the vocal cords and then inserts a plastic tube. This tube can then be connected to a ventilator machine that will breathe for the child. The children in the previous chapters also had plastic breathing tubes placed into their tracheas at various times, although their tubes entered their windpipe through their mouths. Called endotracheal tubes, they can be used for a month or two to connect a child to a mechanical ventilator. If they are left in place much longer than that, however, they tend to cause tissue damage. In contrast, a tracheostomy tube can be left in place for months or even years.

Since a child with spinal muscular atrophy will never again breathe on his own the procedure to place them on a ventilator for the long term would have to be a tracheostomy. This condition does not allow a child to eat either because he or she is too weak to swallow. To solve this problem, a gastrostomy is perfomed where a tube is placed through the child's abdominal wall into his stomach to give liquid feedings. Like the tracheostomy, the gastrostomy can safely remain in place for years.

We can do these things to keep children like Cody alive. The question is: should we do them, and who decides if we will? Until recently there was only one course of action for a child born with the severe, infantile form of spinal muscular atrophy: keep the child as comfortable as possible until he or she became too weak to breathe and cough effectively and died from aspiration pneumonia or simple respiratory failure–not enough oxygen in the bloodstream. Technology has changed this situation profoundly, because when simple in-home ventilators became available for infants and small children, some, but by no means all, began to undergo tracheostomies and gastrostomies. This course of action inevitably led a child in total paralysis, a fully aware brain imprisoned in a body unable to move but still able to feel all kinds of pain and discomfort. These two management pathways–full life support technology versus none at all–stand in stark contrast to one another. Both are presently in use across America. How can these two opposites both be ethical? And how exactly do they figure into Cody's case?

Ethical questions in the PICU often require the balancing of two points of view which tend toward opposite results. These viewpoints have deep roots in our culture. The younger of the two, at least as a formal doctrine, is the utilitarian tradition, exemplified by the writings of the nineteenth century English philosophers Jeremy Bentham and John Stuart Mill. The utilitarian perspective allows that the same action may be ethically correct in one situation but not in another. What is most important is the result of the action; that is, are the consequences good or bad? This way of examining actions ultimately tends toward the conclusion that ethical behavior is that which produces the most good for the most persons.

Even though the philosophical underpinnings of utilitarianism are young, its practice is quite old. For example, various traditional tribal cultures followed these precepts when they reserved scarce food supplies for the young; elderly members of the group did without, even if this caused them discomfort or death. The utilitarian goal dictated that scarce resources should go for insuring the health of those who would carry on the group's existence.

The ethical counterweight to pure utilitarianism is the absolutist viewpoint. All of us would agree that there are some acts, such as cold-blooded murder, which are always unethical no matter the perceived good that may derive from them. These acts are forbidden because they are evil in themselves, even if the person doing them believes that good will result. Ends do not always justify means. This absolutist viewpoint reminds us that actions have an intrinsic moral worth that is independent of their consequences. In the PICU we frequently encounter tension produced by the tug-of-war between these two traditions. Cody's situation was one such example of this inherent tension.

So what are the accepted principles of medical ethics? Medical ethicists generally recognize four main principles: beneficence, nonmaleficence, autonomy, and justice.

The first of these principles, beneficence, is the straightforward imperative that whatever we do should, before all else, benefit the patient. At first glance this seems to be an obvious statement. Why would we do anything that does not help the patient? In reality, we in the PICU are frequently tempted to do (or asked to do by families or other physicians) things that are of marginal or even no benefit to the patient. Common examples include a request for a treatment that the intensivist does not think will help, such as an antibiotic medication, or for a test, such as an x-ray, that the intensivist does not think is needed. Families ask for this sort of thing all of the time. It is so common that, when physicians agree to such requests, we often say that we are treating the family rather than the patient. But is that a bad thing? Is it wrong to treat the family as well as the patient? The answer depends, of course, upon the nature of the requested test or treatment. And that leads us directly to the second principle of ethical behavior in the PICU, nonmaleficence.

There is a long tradition in medicine, one encapsulated in the Latin phrase *primum non nocere* ("first do no harm"), which admonishes physicians to avoid harming our patients. This is the principle of nonmaleficence. Again, this seems obvious. Why would we do anything to harm our patients? But let us consider the example of requests from family members for treatments or tests that the physician does not think will help the child. It is one thing when a family asks me to mix an innocuous herbal remedy in with the child's feeding formula. It is quite another when a family asks me to give a child dying from terminal cancer a highly toxic drug which will not help treat the cancer, and which will cause the child additional pain and suffering. These are easy examples. Much of the time the situation is far murkier.

Pediatric intensivists wrestle daily with the conflicts between the ethical principles of beneficence and nonmaleficence. We have different ways of describing the interactions between them, but we often speak of the "risk benefit ratio." Simply put: Is the expected or potential benefit to the patient worth the risk that the contemplated test, treatment, or procedure will carry? There is often a feeling among families and physicians that doing something, anything, is better than doing nothing. Yet that is not always true. At times it is safer for the patient if we wait a while and see what happens without doing anything, a therapeutic approach we often call "giving the patient some tincture of time." There is a temptation in the PICU, since we do perform quite a few tests on patients, to do a test even though we will not do anything with the information that the test will give us. Yet since no test is completely without risk, mere curiosity is not a sufficient reason.

Our daily discussions in the PICU about the proper action to take, and particularly about who should decide, often lead us directly to the third key principle of medical ethics, which is autonomy. This principle is central to Cody's situation. Autonomy means that physicians should respect a patient's wishes regarding what medical care he or she wants to receive. That is, as much as possible, we should involve the patient in medical decision-making. Years ago patients tended to believe, along with their physicians, that the doctor always knew best. The world has changed since that time, and today patients have become much more involved in decisions regarding their care. This is generally a good thing. Recent legal decisions have emphasized the principle that patients who are fully competent mentally may choose to ignore medical advice and do (or not do) to their own bodies as they wish.

The issue of autonomy becomes much more complicated in the cases of children like Cody, or in the situation of an adult who is not able to decide things for himself. Who decides what to do? In the PICU, the principle of autonomy generally applies to the wishes of the family for their child, although, as you will read in chapter six, we do try whenever possible to determine what the child wants. But what if the family cannot decide what they want for their child? This can happen when there is dissension among family members about the best thing to do, or when the onset of the child's illness or injury has been so sudden and unexpected that the family is paralyzed by the shock of what has happened and is unable to decide anything. What if the child's condition is so critical that there is no time to resolve these issues? Who decides what to do? Finally, what if the child does not want what his or her parents want—at what age and to what extent should we honor the child's wishes?

One can easily see how the principles of beneficence, nonmaleficence and autonomy, notions which, at first glance seem so straightforward,
can weave themselves together into tangled knot of conflicting opinions
and desires. As you will read, this was certainly the case with Cody. The
fourth key principle of medical ethics, that of justice, stands somewhat apart
from the other three. Justice means that physicians are obligated to treat
every patient the same, irrespective of age, race, sex, personality, income, or
insurance status. Up to this point I have been discussing ethical abstractions.
Now it is time to return to Cody's story—to the practical, bedside ethics that
I wrote about in the beginning of this chapter.

When Cody arrived in the PICU he was certainly weak, but not so
weak that he could not breathe at all. We were able to help his coughing
by tapping on his chest to loosen the mucous and then using a suction
device to remove a fair amount of the mucous that he could not cough out
of his airway. We gave him extra oxygen to breathe through some soft plastic prongs placed in his nostrils. Antibiotics helped the infection in his lungs,
his pneumonia. All of these things gave us and his family some badly
needed time to decide what was best for Cody. As a practical matter, we
could postpone when we would need to decide about a mechanical ventilator.

Cody was more than just weak, however. He was emaciated, just
skin and bones, having lost so much weight from his inability to feed
that he weighed only slightly more than he had at birth. He was too
weak to swallow effectively. Although the long-term solution to this
problem is the gastrostomy procedure that I described previously, the
short-term solution is to pass a thin plastic tube through his nose and
down into his stomach, like the one that Tiffany had in the previous
chapter, and use it to feed him. This also would buy us some time by giving Cody the fluid and nutrition that he needed while his parents
decided what they wanted for their child.

All of these things—the oxygen, suctioning of his airway, and passing the feeding tube—improved Cody's situation significantly. By the following morning Cody's lungs were less clogged with mucous, he
needed less oxygen, and the tube through his nose gave him needed fluids and nutrition so he did not appear so dehydrated. The day after that
Cody even seemed a bit stronger, although we knew that this slight

improvement would not last. It was time for his parents to make a true life and death decision.

Steve and Karen were young—Steve was twenty, Karen nineteen. Cody was their only child and they had married when Karen was about six months pregnant. They lived with Karen's parents, although they were just about to move into an apartment of their own when Cody became sick. Steve had just gotten a job, and Karen planned to go back to work when Cody was about a year old. I met Karen's parents, Cody's grandparents, the evening of Cody's admission to the PICU. It was clear to me and to all of the PICU staff that Karen's parents were the decision makers in the family. Karen had never lived outside of her parents' household, and she was used to deferring to their wishes. Steve's parents did not live nearby, and Steve told me that he had been "thrown out of the house" several years before he had met Karen. He had called his parents on the telephone, but he did not expect that they would come to visit Cody in the hospital.

I sat down with Steve, Karen, and Karen's parents the evening that Cody arrived in the PICU to talk with them about what I thought was wrong with the child. I told them about what we could do to improve Cody's lungs and to feed him, but I was quite honest with them in my impression about what the underlying problem probably was. There was really little else that it could be besides severe spinal muscular atrophy, but we would need the blood test to confirm my suspicions. I also told them that I would ask one of the pediatric neurologists, experts in disorders of the brain and nervous system, to see Cody the next day. I suggested that we postpone discussions about what to do in the long-term at least until the neurologist had had a chance to examine Cody.

The talk with Cody's family did not go well, and it was clear to me that, whatever the final decisions were, there would likely be a certain amount of controversy and conflict. Since I am often the bearer of bad news, I do not expect families to like me. Families understandably direct their anger at the intensivist, especially if the bad news is unexpected.

Karen's parents, particularly her father, were very angry at the situation. Although Cody was clearly more comfortable after receiving oxygen, fluids, and suctioning of his airway, they wanted me to immediately summon the neurologist. Barring that, Karen's father wanted to arrange immediate, late-night transfer by helicopter to another children's hospital. I pointed out that we were providing for Cody what he needed at the moment and I also told him that, because of Cody's tenuous breathing situation, it would be unsafe to transfer him to another hospital. The next morning the neurologist came to examine Cody. Even though the blood test had not come back yet, he was quite certain that Cody had severe spinal muscular atrophy, Werdnig-Hoffman disease, and he told this to Karen, Steve, and Karen's parents. When the test confirmed the diagnosis, it truly was decision time.

All of this brings us to a dilemma many families may face in such a hopeless situation: the ethical issue of quality of life. Is life itself always the greatest good, or are there some things worse than death? Most importantly, are there times when the act of prolonging life is itself unnatural? We often phrase this last question another way in the PICU: are there times when our medical care is not in any way healing the child, but merely prolonging the natural dying process? I mean to use the word healing very broadly here, for there certainly are times when, although our specific medical treatments are of minimal use, we still can offer other sorts of care that can be of comfort to the child. Feelings run high on this issue, and many persons hold passionate convictions on the question, even though they may have had little or no personal experience in dealing with what "quality of life" means.

I am not a certified expert in medical ethics. But like most of my pediatric intensivist colleagues, I consider myself to be a type of *de facto* practicing ethicist because I am compelled to make day-to-day decisions that have far-reaching ethical implications. The issue is particularly complex for us in the PICU because much of the discussion of quality of life involves children who cannot always express what they want from life in the same way adult patients can. One of the four basic principles of medical ethics, autonomy, presumes that patients should be able to do to their own bodies what they wish, even if it is not what their doctors advise. In the PICU, of course, we are dealing with what families want for their children. This is a different thing entirely.

Many would say that the very notion of quality of life is inherently subjective because we have no objective standards. Thus, when families are making judgments about the quality of their children's lives, they are really using their own personal criteria. Can this provide a rational basis for ethical decision-making? Most importantly, can families' use of quality of life criteria protect patients like Cody from decisions made simply for economic or social expediency? Bluntly put, how do we prevent the loose application of quality of life standards from leading to instances of outright euthanasia? Medical ethicists vigorously debate these questions and often disagree because, at root, there are no correct answers. Even so, I find one notion to be particularly useful as I ponder the situations of individual patients like Cody: what is important is not the value of Cody's life to others (such as to his family), but rather the quality of his life as he actually lives it. Seen this way, such things as whether a child is in constant, intractable pain or in a permanent coma matter a great deal.

Recent medical history provides us with several profound cautionary tales about the dangers of using assumed quality of life criteria for making life and death decisions. One of these tales is the way in which attitudes toward children with Down syndrome have changed over the past decades. This disorder is a common one. Most readers will have met someone with the syndrome, since it occurs about once in every six hundred births. In its usual form, patients with Down syndrome have a complete extra copy of one of the normal human chromosomes–chromosome 21. This extra genetic material causes a constellation of malformations of the body, although the precise way that the extra chromosome does this remains unknown. The most significant of these malformations involve the heart and the gastrointestinal tract. Surgeons can generally repair these malformations quite easily. Without surgical repair, however, the child with Down syndrome would often die as a consequence, either early (with intestinal malformations) or later in childhood (with heart malformations). Patients with Down syndrome are also mentally subnormal, although the degree of their mental disability is quite variable, and some adults with the disorder can live independently.

At one time, perhaps fifty years ago or so, parents of children with Down syndrome were often advised by their physicians not to request corrective surgery for the malformations. In fact, sometimes families were not even offered surgery as an option for their children. I can remember that time. When I was a pediatric resident, I occasionally encountered teenagers with Down syndrome and unrepaired heart malformations, defects which were by then too far advanced to fix. Parents of these children sometimes told me that they had never even been given the option of cardiac surgery for their children; their child's physician had, in effect, preempted the parents' choices.

It was not only physicians who allowed assumptions about what quality of life meant to affect their treatment of children with Down syndrome; parents occasionally did the same thing. A baby, born twenty-five years ago with the syndrome and named Infant Doe to maintain anonymity during legal arguments, died at six days of age when the baby's parents refused to authorize surgery to correct a problem with the child's intestinal tract. The case caused an uproar, and Congress intervened in the situation with a law that was intended to prevent such things from occurring in the future, at least to infants with moderate disabilities such as Down syndrome. However, like most attempts to legislate answers to difficult ethical questions, the so-called "Baby Doe" law was not helpful as a guide for how we should resolve most of the complicated ethical dilemmas that face us in the PICU.

We must assume that parents who withhold corrective surgery from their children are, in their view, acting in the interests of the children. But what this law really meant was that rather than considering the quality of life of the patient as he or she actually lived it, these decision-makers essentially valued the child's condition as it affected others. In fact, patients with Down syndrome, although typically limited by their mental capacity and occasionally by the medical problems associated with the syndrome, are completely capable of living full and happy lives. In other words, patients with the syndrome are as likely as are you and I to enjoy life and to give joy to others. The example of Down syndrome shows how careful we must be in using presumed quality of life criteria to guide our ethical decisions in medicine.

Sometimes our generalizations, how we cast our language and frame the discussion, get in the way of understanding what it is that we are talking about. One of these concepts is of the importance of doing what is natural, of not going against nature. In the PICU we often grapple with the notion of what is natural and unnatural as being the distinction between truly saving lives and simply postponing death in hopeless situations. In Cody's case, what is "natural" is clear; before high-tech life support systems became available, the "natural" thing to happen was for them to die of aspiration pneumonia before they were just months old. Of course modern medicine in general and high-tech life support in particular are founded on the notion of doing the "unnatural." After all, one hundred years ago, "letting nature take its course" meant children were dying from such varied diseases as tuberculosis, dehydration, and congenital heart disease. We can cure all of these things now. So for Cody we need to frame the question a little differently. Could our principles of medical ethics help his family decide what to do?

For those families in this heart-wrenching predicament, recognizing the first principle of beneficence—whatever we do must, before all others, benefit the patient—is as important to them as well as to physicians. For Cody, this "benefit" would include anything that would calm his anxiety, ease his pain, satisfy his hunger, and quench his thirst. Beyond those things, for Cody the ethical notion of beneficence hinges upon what value we place on simple existence, of being alive. There is no treatment that can improve the state of his underlying disease. If his parents were to choose to place him on full life-support forever, we likely would never fully know his degree of self-awareness. Without enormous effort by his family, and perhaps in spite of it, Cody would be a spectator to life around him, not a participant. Even so, some families choose to attempt that effort.

Although we cannot assume what a child's mental state would be like once he or she were on continuous life-support machinery, we do know what his or her physical existence would be. Children with this disorder, even though they cannot move, have normal sensory nervous systems. This means that they feel everything. If someone inadvertently places them in a bed or a chair with an arm or leg twisted or pinched, they feel it. If their bedridden state causes irritation and sores on their skin, they feel the pain of those sores. They feel these discomforts, but they can do nothing to relieve them because they cannot move or speak. Still, some families choose to do their best to anticipate these things and strive to keep their child comfortable. By doing so, they have decided that mere existence is, in itself, a positive benefit for their child. They have decided that all of the life support systems and the surgical operations needed to maintain that existence—the gastrostomy for the feeding tube, the tracheostomy for the breathing tube, plus the inevitable revisions of those procedures–meet the ethical test of beneficence.

The second ethical principle for parents and physicians to consider is nonmaleficence—nothing we do should harm the child. Some harmful things, such as pain and suffering, are easy to identify; we never want to cause pain and suffering. Never, that is, unless we believe that short-term discomfort is necessary to obtain a long-term benefit; then we will allow it. For a child like Cody, if he were on full life-support, it would almost certainly cause him both physical and mental anguish. What long-term benefit, other than continued existence, would this suffering bring to Cody? If his family were to choose full life-support measures for him, they would be deciding that the intrinsic value of such an existence outweighs the suffering that would come with it. If the benefit were not worth the pain, then this choice would violate the ethical principle of nonmaleficence.

The third key principle of medical ethics is autonomy, the right of a patient to do what he wishes to his own body, no matter what the doctors advise. For children, this decision rests with the family; they will make up their own minds about what is best for their child. Parents should be aware that this inevitably causes conflicts between families and the PICU staff, and among family members themselves. In general, I cannot do things against the wishes of parents, but they also cannot compel me to act unethically. There are procedures to follow when a family and the doctors are at an impasse, and you will read more of these in a later chapter. For Cody, the ethical principle of autonomy means that Karen and Steve could make up their own minds about what to do because our current practice for treating such children is not uniform; people may have strong opinions about what is right, but there are several accepted courses of action. So in this case, the principle of autonomy effectively trumps the other principles. What would Cody's parents decide was best for the child?

Cody's grandfather spent a considerable amount of time researching spinal muscular atrophy and similar degenerative neuromuscular diseases that occur in adults. He was particularly interested in cases of severe amyotrophic lateral sclerosis (ALS), or Lou Gehrig's disease. This is a different disease entirely from what Cody had, spinal muscular atrophy, although

ALS also causes patients to have a progressive weakness that eventually prevents them from breathing until they ultimately die of pneumonia or respiratory failure. Some patients with ALS choose to have tracheostomies and gastrostomies, even though they also eventually become totally unable to move. Stephen Hawking, the noted astrophysicist, is an example of such a patient. Hawking continues to live a full and productive life in spite of his paralysis and constant need for a mechanical ventilator.

Cody's grandfather was an energetic and forceful man, accustomed to getting what he wanted. He was convinced that Cody should receive all of the high-tech PICU support necessary to keep the child alive. He had several reasons for wanting this, most of which were based upon his great faith in the power of technology and biomedical research. He was confident that, sooner or later, medical scientists would find effective treatment for spinal muscular atrophy. Barring that, he was certain that continued progress in medical technology, such as mechanical ventilators, would make the life-support systems that Cody needed to live much less burdensome. He deeply believed that it was wrong to deny Cody the chance to benefit from these future discoveries, marvels which he knew would come.

Cody's parents had not yet decided what they wanted for their son. As the days passed, it was clear to all of us that serious conflicts were building in the family. Most of the tension was between Steve and Cody's grandfather, who believed that Cody should have the surgeries necessary to place him on life support machinery. More than that, he believed that it was morally wrong not to do these things. To him, that would be the same as denying the child needed life-saving measures. We could keep the child alive, and so we should— it was as simple as that.

The physical circumstances of the family also contributed to the building tension. Cody's parents were young, this was their only child, and they were currently living with Cody's mother's parents. They were quite dependent financially upon the grandparents, and Karen also had a close emotional bond with her mother. Complicating matters further was the fact that the grandparents had originally opposed their daughter's marriage to Cody's father, and had only reluctantly accepted it when it was clear that it would happen anyway.

Ironically, Cody's birth had initially defused a great deal of tension in the household. The infant was the only grandchild in the family, and his arrival had immediately focused everyone's energy on him and thereby reduced much of the conflict. Even though Steve and Karen had plans to move into their own home within a few months, Cody's grandparents had spent a great deal of effort in renovating a spare room in the house into a nursery for the new baby. Then Cody got sick, and the tension and conflict returned.

It is no surprise that families of children born with severe congenital problems sometimes experience emotional difficulties revolving around notions of guilt and blame. In such a situation it is perhaps inevitable for parents not to wonder what they might have done to cause the problem, or not done to prevent it. This is a particular issue for children born with ill-defined or poorly understood conditions; often the doctors just do not know what happened to cause the problem. In Cody's case, at least we had a definite diagnosis for his terrible weakness. Even though medical scientists do not understand the precise reasons that the cells in Cody's developing nervous system behaved abnormally, we do know that it is the result of an identifiable malfunction in a specific gene. That defect is originally caused by a random mutation in the gene, an event on the molecular level over which the parents have no control. This was an important thing for Karen to hear from us, because she had become quite distraught over a few whispered accusations from a distant aunt that Cody's disease could have been prevented if Karen had "followed a proper diet and gotten proper exercise."

By this time Cody had been in the PICU about ten days. His breathing problems had improved his first few days there, but he inevitably grew weaker by the day. Cody progressively worsened, and he was rapidly reaching the point where he would need an artificial airway to stay alive. His family needed to decide what they wanted for him.

Although we always want families to consider life and death decisions such as this carefully, postponing difficult decisions can be especially cruel to both children and their families. This is because of the nature of the PICU; sudden crises happen and we must be prepared for them when they do. Children like Cody, those in a very precarious situation, tend to deteriorate suddenly. For Cody, this would most likely take the form of a sudden and complete blockage of the breathing tubes within his lungs with mucous. This would represent a crisis that I would need to solve immediately, within several minutes at most. What if Karen and Steve had not yet decided what they wanted? How could I stand over Cody, breathing tube and laryngoscope in hand, and demand that they decide *this instant* what they want me to do? It is too much to ask of anyone, and it was the reason that we needed to have a plan of action (or inaction) if and when such a thing happened.

Cody's parents needed to make a decision soon, but Steve was still at odds with Karen's grandfather. Karen had not yet really told anyone what she was thinking, partly because she was reluctant to disagree with her father. As it happened, I was able to have a long talk alone with both Steve and Karen about their dilemma.

Steve asked me what I would do if I were in his shoes, if I were Cody's father. This is a question that parents occasionally put to me in difficult situations like this. I rarely answer it, at least directly. Most of my intensivist colleagues do the same. This is not because we are ethical relativists; most of us have strong opinions about which PICU choices are right and which are wrong. But we also recognize that the same decision can be right for one family and wrong for another. We try not to influence a family one way or another simply because of our personal opinions.

When put in this heart-wrenching situation, nearly all parents make excellent ethical choices about what to do. I have also found that when parents make choices that to me seem unwise, it is almost always because they do not fully understand the situation and do not have all the correct information. It is my job to provide that information. That is why it was so important for me to talk with Steve and Karen. I needed to understand what their perceptions were of Cody's life on permanent life-support, and I especially needed to understand what their feelings and fears were about the alternative prospect of watching him die if we decided to do nothing more for him. Altogether, we talked for nearly two hours that night. When we were finished, both Karen and Steve had clearly decided what they wanted: they did not want the surgeries for Cody. This meant that Cody was unlikely to live more than a few weeks. Even though they had decided, they were both very concerned about convincing Karen's father that their decision was the right one.

Families do not always agree about what is best for their child. If the father and mother disagree with each other, then we are at an impasse until the issue is settled. We do have ways of resolving the issue, and you will read more of how we do this in chapter six. In Cody's case, the ethical principle of autonomy speaks clearly: Karen and Steve had the absolute right to decide what to do. Karen's father had his opinion, but he had no right to make any decisions on Cody's behalf. All of us knew that Cody's grandfather would try to change their minds, and that his efforts to do so could upset everyone. The PICU staff was understandably nervous about what the next day would bring.

Cody's grandfather did indeed try to change Karen's and Steve's minds. The way that he did this, however, was to offer a sort of compromise when we all sat down to discuss the situation the next day. He was a skilled negotiator in his business affairs, and he took a standard approach for someone with his perspective—he proposed a solution that, in his view, gave everyone a bit of what they wanted. He proposed that Cody undergo the surgeries, be placed on the life-support systems, and go home (to the grandparents' house) with the nearly around-the-clock skilled nursing care that he would need. The grandfather would have Cody's room extensively renovated to facilitate the child's nursing care. Then, after one year, the family would reassess the situation and reexamine the possibility of taking Cody off his life-support systems, thereby allowing the child to die.

This proposal made sense to a businessman. It might even make some abstract sense to a medical ethicist since there is no ethical difference between never starting a therapy and making a decision to discontinue it after it has been begun. Initiating a treatment does not mean that we must continue it forever; we can always reconsider the situation and stop the treatment. Yet even though this proposal made sense in the abstract, Steve immediately grasped the chief problem with it: Cody would fundamentally not be the same person in a year's time that he was now.

Steve and Karen were not valuing Cody's life as an infant less than his projected life at one year of age. However, Steve pointed out to his father-in-law that it would be especially cruel to allow a child to die who was fully aware of his surroundings and of his family, and who had experienced some aspects of life, even if he were severely handicapped by his paralysis. Steve realized, as all of us did who heard the proposal, that the grandfather was well aware of this dimension. What he really expected was that no one, after caring for a child like Cody for a year, could simply remove the child from life-support at the end of that time. So the compromise really wasn't one at all. The meeting did not end very well. Karen's father was initially disappointed then became progressively angrier when it was clear that Steve and Karen were sticking to their wishes for Cody. The situation was made even more difficult by the fact that the couple was still living under his roof. By the next morning, however, Karen's father had reconsidered his situation. After all, he really did want what was best for his family, as most of us do. He had come to realize that decisions of medical ethics differed in fundamental ways from business decisions. Karen and Steve had spent the night at Cody's bedside, and her father came the next day to say that he would honor the couple's wishes for their son. He only asked that Cody be allowed to die in the hospital, since he could not face taking the infant to his house to die there.

The next morning Steve asked me again what I would do if Cody were my son. This time I answered him: I would do as Steve and Karen had done. On the other hand, I have cared for children whose parents made a different, deeply-considered choice, that of perpetual life-support technology. Even though I would not have chosen that course for my own child, I respected their right to make it for their own child. That is the ethical principle of autonomy in action.

Families faced with such an enormous choice should take solace in the fact that given compassionate support and good information, they will meet the challenge and make the right decision for their child. Even if I could do nothing for Cody's disease, I could help his family meet that challenge. Cody died four days later in Karen's arms, surrounded by his entire family.

CRUCIAL ADVICE FOR PARENTS

Keep a careful eye on your infant and monitor normal progressive movements. At three to four months, for example, a healthy baby will be turning over in his crib.

Again, familiarize yourself with your child's condition; know what can and cannot be done as far as medical treatment is concerned.

Be acquainted with the four ethical principles that guide all physicians; this may help you understand why certain procedures are being preformed for your child or, perhaps, *not* being performed.

As hard as it may seem, try to sort out quality-of-life issues. What are your personally-held beliefs on the subject? What would you do for your child if faced with a life-threatening situation? Some parents find it helpful to consult with a spiritual or religious person on these matters.

Know your legal rights. You are the best advocate for your child.

Realize that it is normal to feel guilt and blame. Be realistic; try not to let these emotions get out of proportion.

Understand the doctor's role as a professional. You may ask his or her personal opinion of what he or she would do, but once informed on all matters, you, as a parent, ultimately know what is best for your child.

Make boundaries clear among family members when dealing with such delicate matters. Parents are ultimately responsible for life and death decisions regarding their child. Other family members, such as well-meaning grandparents, have no legal right to these decisions unless otherwise legally bound.

Chapter 5

Whom Shall We Cure?

Modern medical technology can perform miracles for those in need. These miracles, however, come at a price. Health care costs in America already consume a far larger portion of our gross domestic product than they do for any other developed nation in the world, and this alarming trend shows no sign of slowing down. Intensive care services account for a good share of this enormous cost. Astronomically high medical bills no doubt affect the lives of children and their families during a crisis. How to confront the challenge of paying for these PICU miracles and some oddities about how America funds health care are the topics of this disturbing chapter.

Hope was a fifteen-year-old girl whose father brought her to a local community health clinic late one evening, just before the clinic was to close. Her case is disturbing as it points up the many deficiencies in our current national health care program. It also brings up the topics of illegal aliens, or undocumented citizens, Medicaid, drugs known as steroids and the miracles they can work (when taken properly), and an autoimmune disease called lupus.

Once in the clinic, her father told the doctor that Hope had been having frequent fevers for the past several months. At first her father assumed that Hope had a cold or some other trivial viral illness. But the child's symptoms just went on and on, and she seemed to be getting worse rather than better. The week prior, these fevers had occurred every night, and they were sometimes as high as 103 degrees. Hope had also felt increasingly tired over the past month or so and had missed a great deal of school. She usually worked several evenings each week in a store at a local shopping mall, but she had been unable to go to work for several weeks because of her fever and fatigue. Hope's father was particularly concerned because it seemed to him that his daughter had probably lost at least ten pounds since the beginning of her illness.

Hope had been a healthy child in the past. Before this she had never been in the hospital for any reason, and had been an active, vigorous child with many friends. Her mother had died of cancer several years before, and Hope's father cared for her and her five-year-old brother. One of Hope's aunts also lived in the home and helped care for the family. She had first come when Hope's mother became ill and had remained since then. Her presence was vital for the household because Hope's father, a construction worker, spent ten hours or more each day at his job.

The doctor in the clinic listened to Hope's story and examined her. It was clear to him that the child had a serious illness, not some passing viral infection. Besides what her father had already told him, the doctor noticed a few other things, most notably a rash on her face and upper arms. The rash was a blotchy red color, with the edges of the blotches having fairly sharp margins. The part of the rash on her face was particularly characteristic of Hope's problem; it formed what is usually called a "butterfly" distribution over her nose and cheeks. The rash gets this name because, taken as a whole, the pattern resembles a butterfly–her red nose was the body of the butterfly and her inflamed cheeks formed the wings.

The doctor ordered several blood and urine tests to help him figure out what was wrong with the child. Some of the results from these tests would be available within several hours, but the key test results would not be ready until the following morning. Hope's father wanted to take her home after the samples were drawn, but the doctor was very worried about how Hope looked; she was very pale, weak, and appeared to be dehydrated. She also had a fever of nearly 104 degrees. The doctor told Hope's father that she needed to go to the hospital, both to complete her tests and to treat her dehydration with intravenous fluids.

When Hope's father heard this he became quite worried and agitated. The family had no health insurance at all and Hope had no regular physician. Hope's father had brought her to the community health center because that clinic used a sliding scale of fees, charging less money to those who had less income. The clinic could do this because it received some financial support from a federal government program to offset the costs of caring for those with no insurance. Hope's father told the doctor that he did not even have enough money to pay for her visit to the health clinic and the tests, and he feared that a hospital bill would likely cost thousands of dollars that he did not have.

The doctor tried to reassure Hope's father that, even though the family had no health insurance, Hope would probably qualify for medical assistance from Medicaid, the government program which pays for children's health care in families with low incomes. Besides, Hope was very sick, and the doctor believed that it would be dangerous to send her home. When he heard that, Hope's father relented and agreed to have the child admitted to the general pediatric ward of our hospital.

It was late in the evening by the time Hope arrived on the pediatric floor. She still had a fever, felt terrible, and had taken in very few liquids. The doctor in the hospital ordered intravenous fluids for her dehydration, as well as medication to treat her fever. Once she was asleep in her hospital room, Hope's father went home to be with his son. He told the nurses that he would return first thing in the morning, even though he was very concerned that his boss at the construction site might be displeased enough over his absence to fire him.

The next morning Hope was feeling much better. Her fever was down, and the intravenous fluids had worked wonders in relieving her overall malaise, which they often do in situations like this. The doctor came in about mid-morning to see Hope and to talk to her and her father about the test results. As the first doctor in the clinic had suspected, Hope had a disease called *systemic lupus erythematosus*, or lupus for short. It is a serious illness. It gets its exotic name from the fact that it is systemic, meaning that it affects the entire body, and causes a diffuse red rash, termed an erythema. The word *lupus* is Latin for wolf; some fanciful observer long ago in medical history thought that the rash on the face, in its severe form, suggested the bite of a wolf. Perhaps the Latin for butterfly would not have sounded sinister enough, and lupus is a sinister disease.

Lupus is an example of a kind of disorder that is relatively common, although less so in children than in adults. It is what we call an autoimmune disease. Other examples of autoimmune diseases are rheumatoid arthritis, multiple sclerosis, and Grave's disease, a kind of thyroid problem. These three examples involve three very different parts of the body–the joints, the nerves, and an endocrine gland. But all three share, with lupus, the characteristic of all autoimmune diseases: the body attacks itself. The normal job of the immune system is to destroy invading microorganisms. In an autoimmune disease, the body attacks its own tissues, perversely making antibodies to destroy normal cells.

In the case of lupus, these "autoantibodies" are aimed at one of the building blocks present in nearly all of the cells of our bodies: deoxyribonucleic acid, or DNA. This is the stuff that our genes are made from, and DNA comprises the blueprint that tells each cell what to do and how to function. As with most autoimmune diseases, we do not know why these autoantibodies to DNA develop in a particular individual. We do know that autoimmune diseases tend to run in families. However, many patients with autoimmune problems have no close relations with similar disorders. This was the case with Hope; her father knew of no one in her family who had ever had such a problem in the past.

There are several signs that show the disease—a high fever and "butterfly" rash strongly suggest it; blood tests that indicate signs of inflammation are another. This is all general, nonspecific information, though, and does not point to lupus as the particular cause. There is one very specific test for lupus. This key test is called the anti–nuclear antibody, or ANA. It looks for the presence of the anti-DNA auto-antibodies in a patient's blood and measures the amount there, if any. Hope's ANA was highly positive, which explained why she was so sick.

Many autoimmune diseases give patients symptoms specific to the organ system that is attacked by the particular autoantibody. Lupus is a bit different because there is DNA in every cell in the body except for some of the cells circulating in the blood. Even so, lupus attacks some organs more than others, and most patients with the disease share a variety of symptoms—among them fever, fatigue, and weight loss—which all stem from the general inflammation that is going on throughout the body. Beyond that, lupus commonly affects the kidneys and the heart, causing them to fail, and often inflames the brain. Many aspects of lupus remain mysterious. For example, it is unknown how the anti-DNA autoantibody causes the characteristic butterfly rash–why it affects primarily the face and why in that pattern.

The morning after Hope came into the hospital the doctor sat down with her and her father to explain what all of this meant—what treatment she would need and what the future held for her. The doctor was quite honest when he told Hope's father that, although there are effective treatments for lupus, each patient is different and it was impossible to predict how many chronic problems Hope would have. He would begin treatment that day, and said that Hope would soon be feeling better. He would also ask a specialist in autoimmune disorders, a rheumatologist, to come and see the child later that day. Although all pediatricians know something about lupus, it is a rare enough disorder to warrant the expertise of a specialist.

That afternoon the rheumatologist confirmed that Hope indeed had lupus, and that it was a fairly severe case. He prescribed several medications to bring the disease under control. The mainstay of Hope's initial treatment was an intravenous steroid, methylprednisolone, a powerful, synthetic version of a naturally-occurring hormone, cortisol, which is made in the adrenal gland. Cortisol is one of the "fight or flight" hormones that our bodies call upon when our systems experience significant stress. It allows us to respond to threats by using our energy reserves, and it enhances the function of several key body systems, particularly the cardiovascular system. Cortisol is also a powerful suppressant of irritation and inflammation of all sorts. This is why steroid cream smeared on poison ivy blisters makes them disappear, and why inhaled steroids calm the inflamed airways in persons with asthma. Injected into a vein, steroids are powerful suppressants of inflammation anywhere in the body. That was why the rheumatologist could be confident that Hope would soon be feeling much better; the intravenous steroid medication would block the inflammation that was causing all of her symptoms.

Steroids often work like magic in the immediate treatment of autoimmune diseases. The first patients who received them, as well as their doctors, called them miracle drugs. The two scientists who discovered them won the Nobel Prize. One of my medical school professors was a colleague of these medical pioneers, and was one of the first physicians to use steroids on patients with autoimmune arthritis. He told us how a woman, crippled by arthritis and confined for years to a wheel-chair, had her disability melt away after only a few days of steroid treatment. She told him that it seemed too good to be true— it was.

The steroid miracle comes with a price, a significant one. The drugs that mimic cortisol's natural actions in the body carry with them major side effects, some of which can be life-threatening. If steroids are used long enough, and in sufficient doses, some or all of these side effects will occur in every single patient. The fundamental reason is that inflammation, besides causing us problems, also has benefits; thus a drug that has the power to eliminate inflammation also has the power to do us serious harm. This is particularly the case with the immune system, the part of our bodies which fights off infection. Because normal immunity is closely linked to the process of inflammation, steroids block normal immune function. The results may be catastrophic for the persons taking the drugs because their bodies can be overwhelmed by serious infections.

In spite of all of these problems, steroids remain one of the most useful class of drugs known. The key in using them is to do so in such a way that their possible side effects are minimized and their potential to do good is maximized. The guiding principle for physicians is to use the most powerful steroids in brief pulses for only as long as is absolutely necessary to control the unwanted inflammation. Steroid-induced suppression of normal immunity takes a while to occur, as do many of the other side effects of the drugs; short treatment courses, typically five to fourteen days, avoid many of these long-term problems.

That was the rheumatologist's plan for Hope: to use high-dose, intravenous steroids for only a few days, and then reduce Hope's dose quickly once her lupus was under control. Patients with lupus often must take prednisone, an oral steroid, for many weeks or more, but the side effects are much less of a problem if the drug is taken in a reduced dose or on alternate days. The ultimate goal is to get the patient entirely off steroids and still keep the lupus quiet, although this is not always possible.

Hope started her intravenous steroids the next afternoon and was making great progress just two days later. Her fevers had disappeared, her appetite had returned, and she felt strong enough to walk around the pediatric ward. Her laboratory tests had improved, too; several of the blood tests indicated the degree of inflammation in her body was now close to normal. Everyone was pleased with her progress, particularly her father. The rheumatologist changed Hope's medication from the intravenous steroid to oral prednisone and began to make plans for discharging the child from the hospital. When she went home a few days later, the rheumatologist gave her father a prescription for prednisone and an appointment to see him in the hospital's clinic in about a week. If Hope continued to do well, it was likely that her doctor could then reduce her steroid dose.

Hope went home, but no one in our facility saw her for another three months, at which time her father brought her back to the emergency department. He said that she had been much worse for about a week. Unlike Hope's last visit to the hospital, this time she needed the PICU. She now had a fever of 104 degrees and was barely conscious. She had a severe rash all over her body, not just on her face. Her blood pressure was extremely high. Her heart function was decreased. Blood tests indicated the extent of inflammation in her body was off the charts. Her urine showed dangerous abnormalities. Taken together, these things all meant that Hope's lupus was totally out of control. Her kidneys were failing, her brain was inflamed, and her heart was struggling—what had happened to Hope?

The answer is a sad one: Her father never filled the prescription for the prednisone because he had no money to buy it. Hope was not covered under any health insurance once she left the hospital. Prednisone is one of the cheapest medications there is, almost cheaper than aspirin. Still, for Hope's father, the choices were between food, rent, and Hope's medicine. Since she seemed to be much better, her father hoped that maybe his daughter would not need any more medicine. He had not taken her to see the rheumatologist in the clinic for the same reason: he knew that he had no money to pay the doctor, and he was fearful about what the doctor would say.

You will read later in the chapter about Hope's experience in the PICU. The immediate challenge for Hope and her father, however, was not a medical one; it was a financial one, a challenge shared by millions of families like hers. How should we pay for the miracles of modern medicine? Further, how can it be that, for lack of the few pennies needed for each prednisone pill, Hope's family instead found themselves faced with thousands and thousands of dollars in PICU bills? What sort of system is this?

In the previous chapters you have seen the technological marvels of the PICU. Hope did not need much technology. Her challenge concerned something else–money. The daily charge to the patient in our hospital just for a PICU room is, at the time of this writing, $2,448. This covers the nursing care and the basic equipment at the child's bedside; all that you get for that sum are monitors, clean linen, and Kleenex. Everything else is extra. For example, a day's use of a mechanical ventilator, which includes the bedside care of the respiratory therapists to run it, is $1,100. These are hospital costs only; professional fees charged to the patient by physicians are separate. Physician charges in the PICU are based upon either the particular procedure he or she does for the patient, the overall time that the physician spends with the patient, or a combination of these things. Physician charges for the first day of a child's stay in the PICU can easily top $3,000, much higher if the child needs any major procedures such as surgery.

Critically ill children admitted to the PICU usually need x-rays and blood tests, all of which are billed individually to the patient. The medications given to the patient, along with all of the intravenous infusion supplies needed to give them, are also billed separately. Adding up all of these charges, a day in the PICU can easily cost around $10,000. Very sick, very complicated children like Robert, the boy in the first chapter, can quickly run up a PICU bill of half a million dollars or more. Why are these costs so high, and who pays these enormous sums?

This book is about people, not the economics of health care. But if you are a parent of a child in a possible PICU situation and little or no health insurance, you need to acquaint yourself with some hard-hitting money matters. Health care costs, after declining somewhat during the middle of the 1990s, are once again increasing faster than the overall rate of inflation. This is an immensely complicated and controversial subject, although most observers agree on a few general points. One reason for the increasing costs is that expensive new technologies and treatments are constantly being introduced into medicine, often without much analysis regarding whether or not they are truly better for the patient than existing, and usually cheaper, methods. American physicians, like most Americans, tend to think that newer is better, so we rush to give our patients the benefit of the latest great thing without much consideration to its cost.

Many observers believe that the skyrocketing cost of medications is driving medical inflation. There is heated debate about whether or not excessive profits by pharmaceutical companies are the main reason, or at least a contributing reason, for the high cost of drugs. True or not, a fundamental reason for the steady increase in the proportion of our medical bills that goes to drugs is that we have experienced a steady increase in conditions that we can now treat with medications. We are, in fact, victims of our own success. Drug therapy was cheap when we hardly had any.

The health insurance coverage among the children admitted to America's PICUs is divided into several large categories: private insurance, which includes many versions of managed care plans; various government programs, the largest of which is Medicaid; and children from families with no health insurance at all. Most observers believe that the last of these three groups is constantly growing, although there is debate about the truth of that assertion as well. What all of these insurance plans are and how they work is a complicated subject. Some would term it an incomprehensible muddle. My goal in this chapter is to explain the workings of health care financing in sufficient detail for parents to understand how it actually affects the care of children like Hope. You cannot really appreciate how chaotic the situation is until you see how it affects children like her.

Traditional health insurance, as that term is generally understood, is rapidly disappearing from the health care scene. It is important to point out, however, that "traditional" in this sense is a relative term. Until the 1930s, most Americans either paid cash for their health care or they went without. Physicians and hospitals provided some charity care for patients who did not have money to pay for services, but they were under no obligation to do so. Insurance companies established health insurance plans as they did their other insurance ventures—participants paid regular premiums to an insurance company in return for having their medical bills paid by the company when they needed health care. The health insurance plans made money for the insurance companies in the same way that life or auto insurance plans made money: the companies invested the premium dollars and pocketed the accrued interest, meanwhile anticipating how much money to keep on hand to pay out claims. Virtually all of these plans covered only hospital care, expecting subscribers to pay for physician office visits themselves. This made sense when most things that were done to patients took place in the hospital. Now, of course, a wide variety of expensive medical encounters take place outside the hospital.

The first health insurance plans generally paid out to physicians and hospitals whatever fees were generally felt to be "reasonable and customary" for the care rendered and did not question too much the details of the bills. In that "fee for service" environment, physicians and hospitals in a particular geographic region usually charged more or less the same price for the same service and neither the insurance plans nor the individual patients could do much in the way of cost comparisons because, until fairly recently, advertising of medical services was considered to be unethical.

It is easy to see how, under this system, there is little constraint on costs other than physician judgment regarding what services are needed. In fact, overuse was encouraged because the more services that physicians and hospitals provided, the more they got paid. Further, since the patient with such an insurance plan paid little or nothing out of pocket for hospital bills beyond a monthly premium (large co-payments were a thing of the future), there was essentially no measure of financial restraint built into the system at the subscriber level. When physicians had relatively few medicines and treatments to offer, this system worked. However, as increasingly expensive treatments and procedures appeared, costs skyrocketed. This is why less than five percent of the children admitted to America's PICUs have insurance coverage of this sort; the risks to the insurance companies are huge, and they have little control over the total cost of the care provided.

Virtually all private insurance now takes the form of some variant of what is termed managed care. In a typical PICU, some sort of managed care plan covers twenty-five percent of the children. The rationale behind managed care is that a significant portion of the exploding costs of medical care can be attributed to the lack of any constraints under traditional insurance plans regarding what insurance would cover. The concept of managed care is that, before various kinds of expensive procedures or treatments could be given to a patient, the need for these treatments must be justified. Some managed care policies decide that specific treatments or procedures are simply not covered in the plan, in effect asserting that they are never justified or that there are always cheaper alternatives that are just as effective. There are many, many variants of how managed care works, and this variability can be extremely frustrating to physicians and hospitals because every insurance carrier has its own set of administrative rules.

Although the managed care plans vary considerably in the details of how they operate, they share one overriding characteristic: they never pay retail. At very frequent intervals, the plans negotiate with physicians and hospitals how much money that they are willing to pay for the care provided to their subscribers and because of their clout they usually obtain deep discounts below "sticker price." These reduced prices benefit the plan members, but they can be extremely unfair to families of children like Hope. The overall result is that children in the PICU receiving similar care may have very dissimilar bills for that care. This is particularly unfair to those families without any insurance at all because, although managed care plans virtually never pay the standard, quoted price for PICU care such as I listed at the beginning of this chapter, individuals with no such influence are billed at the going rate for the care. So those unfortunate families with no health insurance get hit for the full price, sums which almost no one can possibly pay, especially if the family was already unable to afford basic health insurance in the first place.

For most PICUs the 800-pound gorilla of health care funding is Medicaid. This is because Medicaid is the largest single insurer of children in America. Last year, for example, more than half of the children in the PICU where I worked were Medicaid patients. So in order to understand who pays for all of the PICU care in America, one needs to understand the basics of what Medicaid is and how it works. It is ironic that, in spite of all of the heated debates in the media about government involvement in health care financing, few seem aware of the fact that the government already pays for the care of at least half of the children in my PICU. Many large urban PICUs have a much higher proportion of Medicaid patients—often three-quarters or more.

The Medicaid program was established in 1965 as Title XIX of the Social Security Act. It was a sort of companion piece of legislation to Medicare, the federal program of health insurance for the elderly, but with important differences. The key difference is that, whereas Medicare is strictly a federal program, Medicaid is a partnership funded jointly between the federal government and the individual states. The relative contributions of the states and the federal government vary from state to state, but for most states the federal portion amounts to just over half of the total bill. Medicaid is an entitlement program, which means that every person who qualifies for the program must be allowed to enroll. In theory, participation by the states in Medicaid is optional. However, all fifty states and the District of Columbia have the program.

The federal government gives the individual states fairly extensive discretion in how they administer the Medicaid program. There are, however, some minimal requirements that the states must follow for eligibility. These are based on income. The groups of individuals that the states are required to cover with Medicaid include pregnant women, infants, children up to age eighteen, and the disabled. Eligibility for Medicaid varies somewhat depending upon what category that person is in. For example, federal law requires that Medicaid cover all pregnant women and children under age six in families with incomes of up to 133 percent of the federal poverty level; for children age six and older, the required federal income threshold for eligibility drops down to 100 percent of the poverty level.

The state where Hope lived is not a generous one for Medicaid. Its eligibility levels for the program were (and remain) the mandated federal minimum, no more: for a pregnant woman or a child under six years of age living in a family of four the threshold is an annual income of $24,472 or less; for children between six and eighteen it is an annual income of less than $18,400, which is the federal poverty level as of this writing. Adults under the age of sixty-five, even if they meet the low income requirement, are not eligible unless they are disabled or pregnant, in which case they may qualify.

Medicaid puts enormous fiscal pressure on the states because, unlike the federal government, most states are required to operate within a balanced budget from year to year. So when the state portion of the Medicaid bills come due, they need to be paid in full from a fairly fixed pot of money. And, since Medicaid is an entitlement, the states have only minimal control over the number of Medicaid participants who need to be cared for with this fixed sum. The states can reduce their pool of eligible persons by enrolling only those who meet the federally-mandated minimums, but they must enroll at least those. Unlike private insurance plans, Medicaid cannot reject a person because he or she has a pre-existing condition that is expensive to care for; Medicaid must enroll all who qualify financially. And it is just this subset of patients–poor children, disabled adults who are unable to work–for whom Medicaid assumes a disproportionate share of the medical care costs.

Medicaid's financial troubles have put an enormous strain on PICUs across America. Just slightly more than twenty percent of the children in the city where Hope and her father lived are enrolled in Medicaid. All things being equal, one would expect that the proportion of PICU patients on Medicaid would parallel the situation in the general population. However, all things are definitely not equal. In fact, the disparity is dramatic. In the year that I cared for Hope, nearly fifty percent of my PICU patients were Medicaid patients. This means that, on average, we had over twice as many children on Medicaid in the PICU than were present in the general population. Why is this? Are children on Medicaid more likely to be critically ill? Is this a situation peculiar to where Hope lived?

That situation actually reflects what is seen in children's hospitals across the country. Children on Medicaid are indeed not just more likely to *land* in a PICU than are children with private insurance, but Medicaid children are more likely simply to *need* admission to a hospital. The National Association of Children's Hospitals reports that nearly fifty percent of all of the children admitted to its member institutions are on Medicaid. There are several possible explanations for this observation, but chief among them is that children on Medicaid find it very difficult to get regular medical care. This is because it is difficult in many areas to find a physician who will take Medicaid patients. The reason is money.

It is generally true that the costs in time and overhead for a typical pediatrician or family physician to see a child on Medicaid for a typical office visit is more than the physician is paid by Medicaid for the visit. In other words, the doctor loses money on every Medicaid patient. Although all of the pediatric practices in the city where Hope lived have some Medicaid patients, one can see that, if the practice has too many children on Medicaid, the doctor will go broke. The result is that pediatric practices across the country are less and less likely to see Medicaid patients. Therefore many children have difficulty obtaining routine medical care. This is a huge issue if the child has a chronic medical problem such as asthma, diabetes, or in Hope's case, lupus. For such children, visits to the doctor to manage their problem are the ounces of prevention which, when regularly applied, can prevent the expensive pounds of cure that are hospital admissions. Yet these children often cannot get the regular care that they need.

Many localities have tried to meet the challenge of providing medical care to children like Hope by establishing community health centers. These facilities are able to care for large numbers of Medicaid patients, as well as for patients with no health care at all, because they are eligible to receive special government grants to offset the costs. Hope's father knew about the local community health center's reduced fees for those who had no insurance, which was why he took his daughter there in the first place. Other towns and cities care for children like Hope at publicly-funded hospitals or other facilities, passing the cost for that care on to the taxpayers. Hope's father was poor, with an income less than the threshold amount that would have qualified his children for Medicaid—why then did he not sign Hope and her brother up for the program? Did he simply not know about Medicaid? The answer is that Hope's situation was complicated by another crucial fact.

I have not used Hope's real name in this chapter, of course. Even so, the pseudonym that I chose for her would have been better given as Esperanza, or Hope in Spanish. Hope was born in Mexico, as were her parents. Her father had first come to the United States when Hope was a baby. At that time he had a valid work permit to do so. The next year he had returned to Mexico to make plans to move his entire family to the United States. He knew that he could never do this legally, so he planned to join the millions of his compatriots who live in this county illegally. So he crossed the border again and made his way to a large city, where he found work and a place to live. His brother later managed to successfully bring Esperanza and her mother across the Mexican border.

The family had since lived in the United States for many years and since had another child, Esperanza's brother, who was the only American citizen in the family. Both Esperanza and her brother went to public school. In spite of his status as either an illegal alien or an undocumented immigrant (depending upon one's politics), Esperanza's father had found no difficulty in obtaining work. He could not, however, enroll his children in Medicaid. He also could not afford health insurance for them, and his employer, who most likely knew of his illegal status, offered none through his job.

Federal law requires that any person who needs emergency medical care and who appears at a licensed hospital must either receive the needed care there, or else be transferred to a facility where he or she can receive it. This requirement applies to everyone, whether or not the person has any money to pay for the care. More important than federal law is the principle of medical ethics that persons in dire need of medical care should receive that care. That is why Esperanza was admitted to the hospital: she desperately needed medical attention. But how could her father ever pay for that care? He had little or no money to do so. In fact, he did not have to pay anything at all. Medicaid paid.

The Medicaid program, at least in Esperanza's state, has an interesting provision. When she was admitted to the hospital, Esperanza qualified for what was called "emergency Medicaid." That term meant that, even though Esperanza did not qualify for Medicaid because of her illegal citizenship status, she received Medicaid status for the duration of the emergency hospitalization. However, once Esperanza left the hospital she again had no health insurance. So her father did not buy the prednisone, and he did not take her to see the rheumatologist. The irony of this situation is that when Esperanza needed hospital care the next time, for her uncontrolled lupus, Medicaid once again gave her "emergency" status and was willing to pay her hospital bills, costs which this time ran to more than fifty thousand dollars for her PICU stay. But this is a book about people, not policy. Let us return to the bedside of a critically ill child.

Esperanza was barely conscious when she arrived in the PICU from the emergency department. She was suffering from several complications of out-of-control lupus. The first of these is termed lupus cerebritis, the latter word simply meaning "inflamed brain" in Latin. This is a serious condition, one which can lead to lasting damage by causing strokes, areas where the brain has not had enough oxygen. I ordered a

CT scan of her head to see if this had already happened; it showed the expected mild brain swelling from the inflammation, but fortunately no strokes—at least not yet.

The lupus was also giving Esperanza kidney failure. This showed itself in several ways. Before I even had any test results back I could see that her blood pressure was dangerously high and that her urine was a rusty color. Within a few hours the tests of her blood chemistries showed, as had been the case with Ronnie in chapter two, that her kidneys were not adequately clearing the waste products from her bloodstream. If this continued, I would need to connect her to the same kind of kidney dialysis machine that I had used with Ronnie. Her kidney problem was also making her whole body retain too much fluid, and her hands, feet, and face were puffy and swollen as Ronnie's had been. This was also why her blood pressure was too high; she had too much fluid in her blood vessels.

Severe lupus often inflames the outer surface of the heart, the pericardium, and this seemed to be happening to Esperanza along with all of the other problems she was having. I suspected that she had this when I heard an extra, unusual sound with each heartbeat (termed a friction rub) through my stethoscope. It suggested that, along with all of the other inflammation going on in her body, Esperanza also had pericarditis—an inflamed pericardium. This can be serious or even life-threatening because the inflammation can interfere with the heart's ability to pump blood normally. The injury can persist for a long time because, as the inflamed pericardium heals, the tissue can scar and constrict the normal motion of the heart as it pumps blood. Two tests of her heart, an electrocardiogram and an echocardiogram, confirmed my suspicion that she had pericarditis.

Altogether, Esperanza was critically ill with inflammation in her head, her heart, and her kidneys, all of which could have been prevented had she been taking less than ten dollars worth of prednisone. Her father was agitated and remorseful that all of this had been, in his opinion, his fault. Yet it was clear that he meant the best for his daughter. His command of English was not good, and her dramatic response and improvement following her first steroid treatments had led him to believe that she really was better, even cured. He had no idea that she could become ill again so quickly.

As things turned out, Esperanza was lucky. Her PICU stay, in comparison with the children you have met in previous chapters, was uneventful. She was desperately ill when she arrived in the PICU, particularly from her brain inflammation, and during her first night in the PICU her coma would worsen and I would need to place her on a mechanical ventilator. She also had a seizure that night. I treated it with a standard anti-seizure medication and she had no further problems of that sort. Her overall inflammation improved after several doses of intravenous steroids. By the next morning she was more alert, although still not clearly herself; by the next day she was mentally back to normal.

In spite of this improvement, she continued to show signs that her lupus "flare," as exacerbations such as this are known, had left her body more damaged than it had been at the time of her first episode. The most obvious of these signs was her rash, which persisted for several more weeks. That was mainly a cosmetic issue. More ominous was the fact that her kidney function had not returned to normal even a month later. This was not a problem at that moment, but it meant she could have poor kidney function for many months, perhaps forever. Chronic kidney disease is common among patients with lupus, and it tends to worsen with time. Many patients who have continued problems of this sort end up needing a kidney transplant years later. It is too soon to tell if this will happen to Esperanza.

What if Esperanza one day needs a kidney transplant—can she have one? At this time, at least in the state where Esperanza lives, the answer is no: she cannot receive a kidney transplant. More than that, she could not receive regular dialysis treatment if her kidneys were to fail, treatment that all kidney failure patients need while they wait for a transplant. So if Esperanza does develop complete kidney failure, she will die from it. She cannot receive these treatments because, as an illegal alien (or undocumented immigrant), she is not eligible to be enrolled in any government health care program that would allow her to see a doctor outside the hospital. The only medical care that she can get is when she appears in the emergency department, again critically ill. Then she will probably once more be admitted to the PICU for weeks of painful, expensive care, again likely to be paid for by Medicaid under the "emergency Medicaid" provision. As you read this, the situation may have

changed for the worse for children like her. As I write, the state legislature is considering various bills to limit or even prohibit children like
Esperanza from ever getting any state-funded care at all. In that case she
would most likely die if her lupus flared again.

Esperanza is not an American citizen. Yet she is here, on our
doorstep, sick with a chronic, serious, and often life-threatening disease.
What should we do with her? Should we just send her, along with her
family, back to Mexico? Should we enroll her in regular Medicaid? If
nothing else, that would spare her the acute suffering from lupus flares,
as well as save Medicaid a large amount of money because she would
stay out of the hospital. I do not know what the answer is to this question. I do know that children just like Esperanza show up in PICUs
across America all of the time. They are not going away; in fact, their
numbers are increasing.

The fundamental question here really is that of what health care
represents: is it a natural right of all citizens, to be paid for by all citizens
through their taxes, or is it a commodity to be purchased like other
commodities only by those who have the money to do so? In other
words, just what is society's responsibility to the individual health care
needs of its citizens, particularly those who cannot afford to purchase
health insurance? The United States is unique among the world's eco-
nomically advanced nations in that we do not provide our citizens with
a universal health care plan of some sort. The great debate about the
proper role of government in health care financing, when viewed from
my perspective in the PICU, is rapidly becoming moot anyway. This is
because, as you have read in this chapter, federal, state, and local governments are already paying the medical bills for most of my patients, and
government's share of PICU costs, planned or not, is steadily growing.

Is emergency, life-saving medical care really a commodity like any
other? Some people think so. This sort of extreme free-market position
may seem reasonable when viewed in the abstract. After all, nothing in
life is free, so we should pay for what we use. However, this viewpoint
is not so reasonable when seen from a child's bedside in the PICU,
where deciding whether or not to use the "commodity" of health care
determines whether or not that child lives or dies. When we purchase a
car we consider costs and whether or not we can afford a particular

make or model. In the PICU, however, neither the physician nor the child's family have the inclination or even much opportunity to consider cost when deciding upon a course of action. Both the family and the PICU physicians typically do what they think is needed and worry about the costs later. Medical ethics, as well as the law, require that we give each child the best and most appropriate care that we can, irrespective of cost. Thus Esperanza, whose father could not afford prednisone in the free marketplace of medical care, could still be legally and ethically entitled to astronomically more expensive care in the PICU.

Such matters are complicated. They are also contentious. Yet money really *does* matter, as shown in a recent study by the Institute of Medicine of the National Academy of Sciences: unexpected bills for health care are the major contributor to half of all personal bankruptcy filings. Medical bills, not frivolous credit card debt, are the leading cause of personal bankruptcy in America.

It is fair to say that most people, no matter what their political slant, believe that America's health care program is inefficient. The public debate often seems to consist of competing voices, each focusing on this or that aspect of the issue. I certainly have no proposal to solve the problem. But this particular story dramatizes how the debate needs to be grounded in what is actually happening at each patient's beside. A major tragedy of the present state of affairs is that, although we often save children's lives, the economics of PICU care can be ruinous to their families.

Esperanza's story puts a challenge to all of us: what can we do, what should we do, when the time comes that we can no longer afford to give every child who appears in the PICU all of the care that they need? If things go on as they are, that time is surely coming.

I do not know what happened to Esperanza. I do not know where she went when she left the hospital—and that was years ago. I hope that her father found the money to at least buy her prednisone. I do know that I never saw her again. Perhaps her family moved to another place, perhaps back to Mexico. Perhaps her lupus went into a long remission and she is well, or perhaps she died. I do not know. Her story and her plight is one of the most troubling to me, and I still do wonder about her.

CRUCIAL ADVICE FOR PARENTS

Know what your current health insurance plan covers and does not cover. If the policy is unclear to you, contact a company representative to help explain specifics.

If you do qualify for Medicaid, find out what the specific plan coverage is for your particular state, as it varies from region to region.

Two helpful websites on government and federal health and medical insurance programs are:
www.cms.hhs.gov and www.childrenshospitals.net.

Lupus is a systemic, auto-immune disease and, as such, means that the body attacks its own tissues instead of destroying invading microorganisms.

Physical signs of the lupus include: fever, fatigue, weight loss, and a "butterfly" rash that appears on the face.

Steroids are often used in the treatment of lupus. Be aware of these powerful synthetics and how they are administered. They can work miracles, but often at a price.

Chapter 6

Knowing When to Quit

PICU technology is a marvelous thing. It saves lives. But it is only a tool, a means to an end, a way of reaching a goal. Sometimes it seems to families in the PICU, and even to the PICU staff, that the technology is in control, dictating what we do, rather than the other way around. It is a challenge at such times to take charge of the situation, to remind ourselves that the technology is only one of several tools we use in the PICU, and for some patients it is the least important one in our toolbox.

This chapter's story is complicated in that it reminds us once again of the paradox of PICU care: In the midst of this amazing and sophisticated hi-tech machinery stands an ultimately most important concept—that of humanistic medical practice. This chapter tells how one patient and her family understood this and met the challenge facing them.

Shelly lived in a small farming community out on the Great Plains. She was an exuberant girl who was one of the sparkplugs for the student body of her small high school. Her greatest challenge came to her in the form of leukemia in her junior year. What follows is a story of a particularly difficult cancer to treat, its ensuing complications, medical ethics, a parent's love, and one girl's amazing, graceful spirit.

Shelly's greatest love was animals, and that is how, as coincidence would have it, I came to meet her long before she appeared in my PICU. Most small towns like Shelly's have active 4H programs, and Shelly was a passionate participant in her local 4H horse program. She and her mare

won enough ribbons and trophies at those horse shows to fill the family living room. I first met her as she was trotting her horse around the
center of the huge central arena at the state fairgrounds. Shelly wanted
to be a veterinarian. With her drive and grade point average, she would
easily have gained admission to her state university's veterinary school.
But instead, during her junior year in high school, Shelly got sick.

Her mother first noticed Shelly's illness when this usually incredibly active child seemed for a month or so to be unusually tired all of the
time. In addition, the child looked pale. Shelly never complained about
anything, so her mother questioned the child about how she was feeling. Shelly told her that she had been bothered for several weeks by
increasingly severe leg pains that had begun to awaken her from sleep.
She had first attributed these pains to muscle strain from basketball practice, but they seemed unrelated to how hard she had exercised. Shelly's
mother was not too worried about this at first. For one thing, Shelly had
never been sick with anything before in her life; for another, Shelly had
been pushing herself very hard lately in preparation for the summer
horse shows. But when things did not get better over the next week, and
when Shelly developed a fine, red rash over her body, her mother took
her to see the doctor.

The family doctor had known Shelly all of her life, having deliv-
ered her when she was born. Once in his office, he noted that Shelly had
a low-grade temperature and had lost about ten pounds since her last
sports physical. The doctor found several other disturbing things when
he examined the child. Besides being clearly pale, Shelly had a rapid
heart rate and a heart murmur, an unusual sound heard with a stethoscope held over the heart. When he felt her abdomen, he found that her
liver and spleen were enlarged and that those organs felt abnormally
firm. The doctor also noted Shelly's rash— tiny bleeding vessels just
beneath the surface of the skin called petechiae. These are caused by an
abnormally low number of platelets, a particle which circulates in the
blood and helps the blood to clot. Without enough platelets, small blood
vessels rupture and bleed, giving rise to the rash.

Concerned, Shelly's doctor sent her over to the local hospital to
get some blood tests done. One of these, a simple test called a complete
blood count and differential count, soon showed what was wrong with

Shelly: she had a form of leukemia, cancer of the blood. The leukemia cells had packed into her liver and spleen, making those organs abnormally large and hard, and were crowding out the normal blood cells from the marrow of her bones, which is why her legs hurt. This same spreading of the cancer in her bone marrow was why her platelet count was so low and why she was so pale-looking and anemic; her bone marrow, where the body's blood cells are made, had nearly stopped making normal blood components–it was only making leukemia cells. The heart murmur heard earlier by the doctor was the result of her heart working that much harder due to the anemia.

Her parents were stunned by the news. Shelly had hardly ever been sick, and now she had a life-threatening cancer. For the next few days her family rode an emotional rollercoaster, alternating between brave resolve and tearful feelings of hopelessness. Shelly herself, who had always worked hard to get what she wanted, reacted as many cancer patients do when they first receive their diagnosis: she believed that with hard work, her cancer could be beaten. The immediate problem for Shelly, however, was that a great deal depended upon precisely what kind of leukemia she had, since different forms of blood cancer in children have quite different responses to treatment. Her family doctor referred Shelly to a pediatric hematologist-oncologist, a pediatric specialist who is an expert in diseases of the blood, particularly the leukemias. The hematologist, who was a colleague of mine, examined Shelly's bone marrow a few days later. He diagnosed the precise kind of cancer that she had to be acute myelogenous leukemia, a particularly difficult leukemia to treat.

The past fifty years have seen a large amount of research devoted to leukemia in children, which has led to major advances in treatment. Hematologists can actually cure some forms of leukemia, although the course spans several years and the drugs used to treat it are dangerously toxic. Unfortunately, Shelly's form of leukemia was not potentially curable if treated with drugs alone. Shelly's only chance for survival was for her hematologist to treat her with a two-stage approach. The first stage was to give Shelly a succession of drugs over several months intended to kill all of the leukemia cells in her body, a process called induction chemotherapy. This experience is brutal to more than the cancer cells; the children undergoing induction for acute myelogenous leukemia can get extremely ill from the drugs and may even die from them. The goal of induction therapy is to get the child into remission, a state in which the hematologist cannot find any evidence at all of the cancer in the child's blood or bone marrow.

But even if a child achieves remission and the hematologist cannot find any cancer cells, we know from experience that, for Shelly's kind of leukemia, a few bad cells are still lurking somewhere in the child's body. In time, the child always relapses. The leukemia then explodes once more into rapid growth, and when it does it is often resistant to the effects of the drugs used to get the child into remission in the first place. A relapse with Shelly's form of leukemia is always fatal. Shelly's only chance for survival was to undergo a bone marrow transplant while she was in remission—and even that might not work.

As things turned out, Shelly successfully achieved remission from her leukemia and then underwent a bone marrow transplant, receiving the transplanted cells from her brother. The blood cells of the donor must match those of the patient in many ways, which is why most marrow transplant patients receive their new cells from a close family member. Bone marrow transplants themselves carry major risks for death, primarily from the side effects of the drugs necessary to prepare the patient's system to receive the transplant. Sometimes the transplant does not work because the newly transplanted cells die off before establishing themselves in the recipient's bone marrow. Sometimes the transplanted cells even turn on the recipient's body and attack it, although this so-called "graft versus host disease" can usually be controlled with medications. Shelly passed through all of these lurking dangers and went home with her new blood cells working fine.

All of this had happened during the end of Shelly's junior year in high school. By the following fall, she was feeling well and was back for her senior year in high school. She had begun to gain back all of the weight that she had lost during her illness and had mostly grown the hair back that all of her cancer treatments had caused to fall out. Her greatest disappointment was having missed the summer horse show season. Shelly was still too sickly to participate in most of her previous activities, but she pleaded with her hematologist to be allowed to ride her horse. He was reluctant to let her because Shelly's new bone marrow was still not making quite enough platelets, the cells that help stop bleeding. She was therefore still prone to excessive bleeding if she fell off the horse and hurt herself. Finally, the two struck a deal: Shelly could ride if she only walked the horse–no trotting, no cantering, and always wearing a helmet. She also busied herself filling out applications for admission to colleges with good preveterinary medicine programs.

In January, about a year after she first became ill, Shelly got sick again. She began to have fevers at night and a mild cough. These symptoms progressively worsened over the next week, so she went to see her hematologist, who ordered a chest x-ray. The x-ray showed that she had some sort of pneumonia, which appeared mild at that time. Even so, her physician admitted Shelly to our hospital. He did this because the possibilities for the kinds of pneumonias that patients like Shelly can get are many, and the consequences of not diagnosing and treating them quickly are serious. Shelly's physician began her on several antibiotics, gave her extra oxygen, and did several tests to discover what the cause of the pneumonia was.

One particular test done was a bronchoscopic biopsy, a procedure which consists of passing a long, flexible tube with a light on the end, called a bronchoscope, through the mouth and down into the lungs, and then using it to obtain a small sample of lung tissue. A procedure such as this can be uncomfortable, painful, or both. Part of my job as an intensivist is to give the child sedative medications when he or she needs to undergo this type of test. Because these medications have the potential for decreasing the child's spontaneous breathing, these procedures are done in the PICU so that we are ready with all of our equipment to support the child's breathing if needed.

So this is when I next saw Shelly, when she came into the PICU to undergo her bronchoscopy. She recalled meeting me at the state fair two years before, and we talked about horses for awhile. She was not really worried about her pneumonia or the upcoming procedure; she was worried that she would not be able to take her horse with her to college because it would be too expensive to board the animal at a barn, and so she was trying to find a school where she could ride. The bronchoscopy went smoothly and I sent her back to her room on the general pediatric ward when she had awakened from her sedatives. The biopsy showed what was wrong: Shelly had pneumonia caused by a fungus called aspergillus.

The aspergillus microorganism is not rare. It is all around us, since it normally lives in the soil, and we frequently inhale its spores, particularly if the soil is stirred up as it is around construction sites. As it turned out, several new houses had recently been built near Shelly's home. The digging of the new basements may well have been the source for her aspergillus. Normal people don't get pneumonia from aspergillus because they have normal immune systems. Shelly, however, was on medication to suppress the normal function of her immune system so that her body would not reject the bone marrow transplant. Hematologists aim to use just enough of these medications to control rejection of the transplant, but not so much that the patient's immune system is dangerously impaired. In practice, this perfect balance is nearly impossible to achieve. Patients taking these medicines are vulnerable to attack from a host of organisms like aspergillus, microbes which are aptly called opportunists because they seize the opportunity to attack the patient when the natural defenses are down.

Shelly's physicians began giving her a medication to treat the aspergillus, and they also reduced the doses of her anti-rejection drugs just a little bit to allow her own immune system to rise up and help to fight the infection. She did well for a week or so; her cough improved, her need for extra oxygen decreased, and her chest x-ray also showed improvement in the pneumonia. I saw her up walking in the hallway near her room on the pediatric ward and she told me that she expected to go home soon. Her energy was back, and she was busy lining up her college interviews. But over the next few days she suffered from some shortness of breath when she walked and an increasing need for extra oxygen. She also began to have nearly daily fevers and a cough. Although these worsening symptoms began fairly insidiously, Shelly began to deteriorate rapidly. One morning her hematologist asked me to see her in her room on the general pediatric ward because he thought that her respiratory distress had reached the point where we might want to bring her into the PICU.

When I went to her room I could immediately see that Shelly was in serious trouble, and her bedside nurse told me that the child had gotten much worse even over the past eight hours. Shelly was sitting bolt upright in bed with a tight-fitting oxygen mask on her face. She was breathing quite hard and fast, so much so that she could barely speak to me. Her pulse was rapid and thready. She had been unable to eat or drink hardly anything since the evening before, and had needed intravenous fluids to keep her from becoming too dehydrated. She was wide-eyed and clearly very frightened. Feeling that you cannot breathe, that someone is smothering you, is one of the most terrifying experiences that anyone can have. Shelly's mother was also in the room and she too looked frightened by how rapidly Shelly's distress had heightened. Neither of them had slept the previous night; Shelly because she was unable to lie down, and her mother because she was afraid to doze off and leave her child alone in her misery.

It was clear to all of us that, unless she improved over the next few hours, Shelly would need a ventilator machine simply to stay alive. The ventilator could breathe for her, of course, but the main issue for us to grapple with was the cause for her worsening respiratory distress. Was the aspergillus getting worse? She had been responding to the treatment. A more ominous possibility was that she had some new problem. Whatever it was, it was moving quickly.

A child who receives a bone marrow transplant, experiences respiratory failure and then needs to be put on a ventilator is, unfortunately, not an uncommon scenario, but it is one that hematologists and intensivists have studied in some detail. Briefly stated, Shelly's chances for survival were not good; in fact, the statistics for patients like her are frightening. Some physicians have even argued that, since the odds are so long, it is unethical to subject patients like Shelly to the very substantial discomfort of mechanical ventilation and PICU care.

I remember one hematologist who specialized in bone marrow transplants telling me, "I don't need you—ever!" In other words, his view was that PICU care for patients like Shelly on a ventilator machine violated two of the basic principles of medical ethics that I described in chapter four: that of beneficence, because it did no good, and that of nonmaleficence, because it caused needless suffering. My own experience in the PICU with children like Shelly has not been quite so dismal, although the mortality rates are high. In this instance, however, I believed that we should offer Shelly and her family PICU care primarily because we had not yet pinpointed the reason for her respiratory distress, and I did not want to declare her case hopeless until we at least knew what was wrong.

At this point I would like parents to pause and consider another key ethical principle which can be somewhat confusing to all involved. That principle is that there is no ethical difference between not starting a therapy and stopping it after it has been initiated. I believe it is a mistake to say that if we place a child like Shelly on a mechanical ventilator we have somehow begun a process that cannot be stopped, and that we are somehow committed to continuing the ventilator no matter what else happens or what new information we discover. This mistaken viewpoint assumes that PICU technology is an all-or-nothing proposition, that the act of beginning treatments compels us to continue them. This is simply not true. Any medical treatment, whether it is a simple antibiotic pill or a complex artificial kidney machine, can be reconsidered and stopped if all concerned–patient, family, and physicians–agree that such a course of action is best for the patient.

I sat down with Shelly and her mother to discuss what to do. It was clear that the child could not go on much longer like this. For one thing, she was breathing so hard that she would likely grow weary of the effort and stop from simple exhaustion within a few hours, even if her lung condition did not get any worse. Left unsaid for the moment was the high likelihood that, if she did not go on a ventilator, she would soon die. It was Shelly herself who, between panting breaths, stated this obvious fact. She also said that she was definitely "not ready to give up and die." Children in situations like this are usually quite direct and concrete, sometimes in ways that make adults cringe. Children also generally want to do what they believe their parents want them to do. Sometimes this presents a problem. Shelly, however, was unusually mature for a seventeen-year-old, and she was clearly making this decision; she was not ready to quit. After I had finished talking to them, Shelly's mother called her father, who was at home with the rest of the family, to discuss what was happening and decide what to do. After she got off the telephone, her mother told me that they wanted Shelly to come into the PICU because they, too, were not ready to give up after coming so far with her treatment.

I have found that most families in this situation make the same decision for exactly those reasons. Moreover, for all of her life Shelly had been a competitive, high-achieving child. Her struggle with cancer was, for her, one more contest to win. Most parents, I am sure, are familiar with this sort of language; disease is an adversary to beat, and our encounter with serious illness is a battle with something foreign, something outside of ourselves. I used to agree. I have since changed my mind, however, regarding life-threatening disease, particularly cancer, and that way of thinking. This is because we must honestly consider the ravages to the body and to the mind that our treatments will cause, and the martial metaphors of battles and weapons sometimes tend to obscure an honest assessment of the costs of what we do. Still, in this case, I supported Shelly's decision.

Once Shelly and her family had decided, we quickly moved her into the PICU. Her mother brought along the many photographs and pictures that Shelly had pinned up on the walls during her weeks of hospitalization. Shelly asked her mother to pin up two of these large photographs where she could easily see them. One was of Shelly taken the previous year when she had been elected Prom Queen by her high school classmates. She had just completed her induction chemotherapy and in the photograph she was gaunt, emaciated, and totally bald, but she was smiling her best horse show smile, with the prom queen crown on her head and a bouquet of roses in her arms. The other image was of her quarter horse mare, head turned toward the camera, mane and tail done up beautifully, and with a best-in-show ribbon pinned to her halter.

It was now time to place Shelly on a mechanical ventilator, a high-risk endeavor in itself, more so than for any of the previous children in this book. Her ability to breathe at that moment and get oxygen into her bloodstream was marginal, and therein was the risk. In addition, Shelly's chronic illness stemmed from at least two systemic diseases of which we knew—her leukemia and her aspergillus pneumonia. This significantly increased her risk for complications after receiving any anesthetic drugs. She was also a young adult, not an infant, and was fully aware of what was happening to her. This meant that I needed to do whatever I could to relieve her very high level of anxiety since that, too, contributes to the risk.

Soon after Shelly arrived in the PICU, I gave her an intravenous drug called midazolam, which relieves anxiety and interferes with the brain's ability to process short-term memory. The drug usually causes even a conscious patient to have little or no memory of recent uncomfortable events. Her breathing actually improved a bit after the midazolam because she was noticeably less anxious. While she was still sitting up, I gave her a drug called ketamine, which is what we term a dissociative anesthetic agent. Depending upon the dose used, ketamine may or may not cause a child to fall asleep, but either way it completely alters a child's perception of reality; the child "dissociates" from the world. Shelly was looking at the picture of her horse at the foot of her bed when the ketamine reached her brain, inducing the vacant stare and the typical roving eye movements that tell me the drug is working. I then quickly laid her flat in bed and gave her a drug that completely paralyzed all of her muscles. This allowed me to see her larynx clearly with the lighted end of the laryngoscope and place the breathing tube in her trachea. The whole process took just a couple of minutes and she came through it just fine. I then connected her breathing tube to the mechanical ventilator. Once she was on the ventilator, I started her on several sedative and pain-killing medications to keep her comfortable and nearly asleep.

Shelly's mother had been at her daughter's side throughout most of the previous year—through the induction therapy, the preparative therapy for transplant, and the bone marrow transplant itself. She had been there to comfort Shelly when the cancer drugs had caused terrible nausea and vomiting and the bone marrow transplant drugs had filled Shelly's mouth with huge sores so that the child could not eat or drink anything. In spite of that, she was shocked to see Shelly in the PICU after I had finished placing her daughter on the ventilator. Besides the breathing tube in her mouth, Shelly had all of the other PICU life-support paraphernalia that you have met before: a tube coming out of her nose to drain her stomach liquids and one out of her bladder to drain her urine, a large intravenous line coming out of her chest just under her collar bone, and another one coming out of the artery in her wrist. Monitor patches were stuck to Shelly's chest and adhesive was plastered to Shelly's face to hold the tubes in place. When she first saw her daughter like that, Shelly's mother wondered aloud if we had made the right decision in going ahead with all of this. Yet by the next day Shelly's mother, like all of the parents that you've met in this book, found the strength to look beyond the tubes as if they were not there.

It was time to try and uncover what was happening. We asked a specialist in infectious diseases, a physician particularly expert in dealing with unusual and opportunistic infections, to see Shelly and offer his advice. For a day or so it was unclear what was going on, although her lung function was steadily worsening. Then the results of a new bronchoscopic biopsy of her lungs showed the problem: Shelly had a new, highly aggressive infection in her body, particularly in her lungs. This infection was from a virus, one called cytomegalovirus, a notorious problem for patients in Shelly's situation. But it was worse than that. An examination of her bone marrow also showed that Shelly had relapsed; her leukemia had come back.

There is no effective treatment for a patient with Shelly's kind of leukemia, who had received a bone marrow transplant, and who had then relapsed with the leukemia. Even though we could give Shelly additional cancer treatment drugs, they would not work for long, if at all. She could not have another bone marrow transplant. Subsequent scans of Shelly's organs showed that the leukemia had rapidly spread everywhere—to her bones, her liver, her spleen. Relapsed leukemia often behaves like this, with explosive growth of the cancer everywhere in the body. Moreover, even without her relapsed leukemia, virtually no patient like Shelly with cytomegalovirus pneumonia ever makes it off the ventilator. What should we do?

That night Shelly's hematologist and I sat down with her parents to talk about everything. We had enough information to decide what to do, although Shelly herself was not there to participate in the discussion. We explained to Shelly's family that we had no further treatments to offer their child. For us to continue PICU care after we had discovered her leukemia relapse and the cause of her respiratory failure would clearly violate the ethical principle of beneficence, because no known treatment could help, and of nonmaleficence, because these same treatments are quite toxic.

Was it unethical from the start for Shelly to come into the PICU? Was the hematologist who had once told me that he never needed me or the PICU for patients like Shelly correct? After all, he had turned out to be right in this case. Shelly's mother asked me this question. Had we been needlessly cruel to her daughter? My answer then and now is that I do not think that it was unethical to have given Shelly a chance, especially with what we knew at the time, even though the statistics told us that her situation was desperate.

One of the important things that I always want parents to understand at a time like this is that there is no hurry. In fact, if a family's decisions seem precipitous to me, I often will ask them to think about things for a few hours at least. This is the point at which PICU care shifts from caring for both the patient and the family to caring primarily for the family. Sometimes in these situations there seems to develop, for reasons unclear to me, a sense of urgency, of the need to make a decision. In fact, there is rarely any hurry in these matters. Moreover, on several occasions in my career I have spoken with a parent whose child had died in the PICU months or even years previously, and who still had lingering doubts about decisions that they had made at the time of their child's death. Should they have waited? Should they have talked to some other doctors? At this point in Shelly's life, although I could do nothing more for her, I could try to care for her family.

It was soon clear to me that Shelly's parents differed in their viewpoints on what we should do. To understand their differences, I need to describe for you our concept of what constitutes futile care. I listed in chapter four the key principles of medical ethics that form the underpinnings of any physician–patient relationship. I noted then that the concepts of beneficence (what we do must be for the good of the patient), nonmaleficence (do no harm to the patient), and autonomy (letting the patient or the family direct what physicians may do to the patient) can seriously conflict with one another. This is particularly true when a child's family wishes us to do something to their child that we, as physicians, either do not think is justified or is frankly dangerous to the child. Autonomy for the patient does not necessarily mean that the patient's family calls all of the shots. In particular, a family cannot compel me to do something that I believe to be medically unethical.

Futile care is an example of such a situation. What this means, at least to a medical ethicist, is that if a child's medical situation is hopeless, continued aggressive PICU care is futile. In such a situation, the parents cannot force me against my medical judgment to continue such treatment. In fact, many argue that it is unethical for me to continue PICU care at all in such situations. That may sound reasonable and simple in an ethics textbook, but in practice it is anything but simple. There is no test for futility of care; what may seem futile to me may appear potentially helpful to another observer.

But let us consider the situation in another light. Shelly was sedated with powerful pain-killing medications. She was in little or no discomfort at all. Most importantly, her father asked me how I knew that the situation was hopeless. I had to answer that my opinion was based upon my own experience, as well as the opinions and research of experts. But, her father replied, none of that necessarily applied to Shelly. Everyone is unique, he said. In addition, her father was a devout Christian. To him, the fact that I had no treatment to offer Shelly did not mean that no treatment existed; there was prayer and there was the possibility of a miracle. In short, he wanted to give prayer and divine intervention time to work. He was not asking me to add any new treatments, just to continue what we were already doing.

Shelly's mother did not agree with her husband about what to do. She had a perspective that I have commonly encountered among practical-minded persons from a farming background. She was no less devout than her husband, but she thought that it was not right to postpone difficult decisions. She had known her husband for twenty-five years and although she respected and shared his faith, she also recognized that he seemed unwilling to look the situation in the eye.

We concluded our discussion about Shelly with a decision that satisfied everyone's concerns at that moment. We agreed to pursue a course of action that is often taken when there is a disagreement among family members: we decided to change nothing for now. To me, this is an entirely appropriate way to proceed, at least in the short run. I have learned over my many years practicing in the PICU to be very, very cautious about declaring a situation to be hopeless. I told her father that I would not add any new treatments. If Shelly's kidneys were to fail, I would not put her on dialysis. That would violate my ethical sense. On the other hand, I would not withdraw any treatments that we were currently giving Shelly because that would violate her father's ethical views.

When I met again with her parents the following afternoon nothing had changed: Shelly still required a high measure of support with the mechanical ventilator, and she still needed frequent transfusions of blood and blood components to correct the severe bleeding problems that her leukemia was causing. She was still deeply sedated with pain-killing medications. Now our discussion focused on a course of action that could accommodate both my ethical precepts and those of Shelly's parents, who continued to differ in their opinions. How long a time was reasonable to wait for some sign of Shelly's recovery and accommodate her father's wishes: another day or two, a week, a month? I agreed to continue doing as we were, largely because my role had moved from being Shelly's doctor to being a physician for her entire family.

Nature often steps into discussions like these and renders all of our human deliberations moot. In fact, few children like Shelly remain stable and unchanging for very long, and often there is nothing we can do to keep such children alive. Shelly was actually quite stable for several days, although her blood tests continued to show that her leukemia was raging out of control and her viral lung infection was also inexorably progressing.

But what did Shelly want? Was there any way to find that out? And what rights does a competent adolescent, a near-adult, have to decide his or her own fate? It was crucial for us to find out, if possible. To do this, I needed to clear away enough of Shelly's sedative-induced mental haze to the point where all of us—her parents, the rest of her family, and I—could speak with her and find out what she wanted. We had been making decisions on behalf of this vibrant, energetic girl; from what I knew of her, I was sure she would have some opinions on what to do.

Over the next day I adjusted Shelly's sedative medications to the point where she could follow simple commands, such as "open your eyes" and "squeeze my hand," and answer simple questions, such as "do you hurt anywhere?" I also looked to some of Shelly's vital signs, particularly her heart rate pattern and her blood pressure, to help me decide if she was in too much pain or anxiety. In some patients, particularly young children, this optimal balance of awareness comes with significant discomfort. In addition, Shelly's very severe lung failure complicated this process. She required high pressures on the mechanical ventilator to get enough oxygen into her bloodstream. Frequently, in situations like Shelly's, reducing the sedation also reduces the efficiency of the mechanical ventilation such that there is insufficient oxygen in the patient's bloodstream for the vital organs, particularly the brain, to work well. Sometimes this limits what I can do with the sedatives. Still, I had to try.

As things turned out, Shelly once again proved to be an astonishingly brave and mature young woman. The morning after I had adjusted her medications, we could all tell from Shelly's face and demeanor that she was quite aware of her surroundings. She could not speak because she had an endotracheal tube in her airway, but she could nod or shake her head. She could even use a marker to write a few words on a whiteboard. She let us know that, although she was moderately uncomfortable from the ventilator and had some bone pain from the cancer, she could tolerate the situation.

Once Shelly could communicate, I let her family describe to her where things stood. They told her about all of the discussions that we were having on her behalf, and what we thought was the best thing to do. The scene in Shelly's room that afternoon still rests in my mind as one of the most moving encounters I have had in my medical career. I particularly recall Shelly's almost surreal calm, a calm that was drug-induced. Even though she could not speak, it was Shelly who was actually comforting her grieving family, rather than the reverse. Her decision was to be taken off the ventilator. She indicated to her father that if a miracle were to happen, it would have happened already. Her father reluctantly, but genuinely, agreed. Once all had been decided, Shelly saw no reason to wait, even though her parents, particularly her father, would have chosen to postpone the moment.

To experience the world of the PICU is to witness the death of a fellow human being. One hundred years ago death happened outside of hospitals and institutions so that most adults had likely witnessed several deaths in their lifetime. Death was a part of the cycle of life in a way that it no longer is. Today it was time for me to help Shelly die, an awe-inspiring privilege.

Everyone who works in intensive care units is familiar with death. For children, a PICU is now the most common place for death to occur. Often a child's death is sudden and unexpected. But occasionally, as with someone like Shelly, we expect a child to die after we withdraw life support. However, I learned long ago never to predict exactly what will happen when we take away life-support machinery and medications. I don't know what will happen. I fully expect that the child will die, but death could come in seconds, hours, or even days. My job is to allow whatever will happen to happen, and to make sure that the child is kept free of pain and anxiety during that time.

Later that evening I took Shelly off the ventilator. Doing this requires us to confront one final issue in medical ethics. Shelly's sedative and pain-killing medications, in high doses, will suppress her breathing reflex. This is why narcotic overdoses can be fatal outside of the hospital setting. If I left Shelly on these medications, how could I be sure once when I removed her from the ventilator that she would not breathe because these medications were in her body? If she then died because she wasn't breathing, wouldn't that really be a form of euthanasia, of "mercy killing," brought on by the drugs?

This question is one that has concerned such varied groups as medical ethicists, state medical licensing boards, patient advocacy groups for the terminally ill, and even the federal drug enforcement agency. How can we balance the legitimate need for patients to receive the pain relief that these drugs can provide, a comfort ethically mandated by thousands of years of medical tradition, with the equally legitimate fear that physicians will overuse them to the point of actually causing premature death? Will an excessive concern by physicians over what could be construed as their indiscriminate prescription of narcotics in fact result in terminally ill patients not receiving adequate pain relief because doctors do not want to be accused of overusing narcotics?

The answer lies in the actual intent of the physician using the medications. For example, if I use narcotics to ease Shelly's pain and other drugs to calm her anxiety during her final moments, which may suppress her breathing reflex and thereby shorten her lifespan by some small increment, then my use of these drugs is ethical. Indeed, it is unethical for me not to use them. However, it would be unethical for me to use doses of these medications that would be sufficient to abolish her breathing entirely, because then my intent would be for her to die as a result of what I have done. Looking at the issue this way may strike some readers as hairsplitting, but it is not. It really is the intent that matters.

Now we have reached the final phase of Shelly's long journey. Physicians vary in how they go about doing what I am about to describe to you. As I noted before, I regard participating in a child's final moments as an honor granted to me by the child and the family. I strive to return the honor by doing it as skillfully and as reverently as I can.

Later that evening, as Shelly's family gathered around her bedside, I began the process of helping Shelly die. I first increased the narcotic infusion going into Shelly's veins to a dose a bit beyond the point where she had been aware and answering questions. I then quickly reduced the rate that Shelly's ventilator was delivering breaths to verify that she was not too sedated to breathe. I then very quickly removed the breathing tube from her mouth, as well as the tube that went through her nose and down into her stomach. This was the first time in weeks that Shelly's family had seen her face not plastered with tape and with tubes sticking from her mouth and nose. Shelly's mother brushed her hair, which had become inevitably grimy and sticky from the child's long ordeal. Shelly's eyes were closed and she continued to breathe in a fairly normal pattern for several minutes. I watched her closely for signs that I needed to adjust her medications—for gasping, coughing, or choking. She did none of these things. She briefly opened her eyes when her mother spoke to her, then closed them again. As her parents held her hands, Shelly began breathing more intermittently and the amount of oxygen in her blood quickly plummeted. Over the next minute, her heart rate slowed and then entered an abnormal rhythm typical for this situation. She then stopped breathing entirely. Shortly afterwards, I could not feel a pulse at her wrist, and I could not hear a heartbeat with my stethoscope on her chest. Barely a year after she had first become ill, Shelly was dead.

Shelly was blessed with a loving and supportive family, one who in the end ultimately respected their daughter's own choices. But what if a family is divided in their opinions, or cannot decide what to do, or wants physicians to do things that the physicians believe to be unwise, unethical, or even illegal? Then what happens?

If the doctors and a family cannot reach an understanding, all hospitals have ethics committees that can be convened to try to mediate a solution to the problem, whether it is an impasse between family members (typically parents) or a conflict between physicians and families. These committees include physicians new to the case (so as not to prejudge the situation), along with nurses, hospital chaplains, and medical social workers. Hospital ethics committees also have members drawn from the local community, persons not connected with the hospital in any way, which supplies an important balance to the committee's discussions. However, ethics committees are advisory only; they cannot order one course of action or another. If families and doctors are still at an impasse, or if either faction does not agree with the advice offered by an ethics committee, there remains only one way to resolve the issue of what to do—the courts.

The case of Terri Schiavo, played out amidst a media circus during the spring of 2005, served to highlight the role of our legal system in making life and death decisions for persons who are not competent to decide these matters for themselves. Schiavo was, in the opinion of the many brain specialists who examined her, in a permanent vegetative state from which she would never awaken. Schiavo's husband, who had remained legally married to her throughout the many years of her illness, asked permission of Florida's courts to remove his wife's feeding tube and allow her to die. He maintained, based upon his knowledge of her desires before she became ill, that this would have been her own wish for herself. Schiavo's parents contested this claim, asserting that their daughter should continue to have full medical support. Multiple levels of Florida's court system found in favor of the husband and authorized the removal of Schiavo's feeding tube. The woman's parents appealed each of these decisions and the case ultimately went to the United States Supreme Court, which declined to intervene. The Florida Legislature, the Congress, the Governor of Florida, and the President all became involved, respectively passing and signing eleventh-hour legislation aiming to overrule the effects of many court decisions. When all of these maneuvers had played out, Schiavo's feeding tube was removed and the woman died.

What can we learn from all of this? What does Terry Schiavo's and Shelly's story mean to families faced with similar critical decisions? It is my opinion that our society appears to be ever more willing to intervene in decisions that are the proper realm of patients and their families. This is a very disturbing trend, because legislation is an extremely blunt instrument for deciding ethical questions. I am not familiar with the details of the Schiavo case and make no judgment about the correctness of either side in the controversy. But the several courts that deliberated over the case for years were familiar with those details, and we should honor their decision. What would have happened if Congress had passed some vague law that demanded that I try a certain experimental treatment on Shelly? What then?

The courts are far from perfect. However, in my career I have encountered the court system several times over cases like Schiavo's, times when physicians and families, or factions within families, could not agree on what was best for a child in the PICU and the question ended up in court. In each of these cases very well-meaning judges spent hours upon hours hearing complicated testimonies and digesting large piles of documents, some of which were so medically technical that the judge was forced to read additional material just to understand them. I believe, in all of these cases, the courts found their way to well-reasoned judgments.

The lesson that Shelly teaches us is that each case is unique in its own way. Circumstances always differ from patient to patient and family to family. The right to decide issues of life and death rests with patients and their families, and no one else. What is actually astonishing is how rarely the courts are asked to intervene in these questions. The simply amazing thing to me is that virtually all families, no matter how dysfunctional, manage to rise magnificently to the challenge to make thoughtful, appropriate, and ethical decisions about their loved ones. America must trust families to continue to do this.

CRUCIAL ADVICE FOR PARENTS

Be mindful of the paradox of PICU care and the fact that humanistic medical treatment is ultimately most important.

Leukemia, cancer of the blood, takes many different forms in children with varying degrees of difficulty and types of treatment.

Remission is a general term for a state of being in cancer patients where there is no evidence of cancer in the cells, blood, or bone marrow, depending on the cancer.

A key medical principle described in this chapter is that there is no ethical difference between *not starting* a therapy and *stopping* that therapy after it has been initiated.

The Terry Schiavo case points to the need for all adults to have a living will. In the case of children, when parents disagree on the life/death decision, a meeting of the minds must occur. In Shelly's case, through the help of doctors, she was able to intervene and sanction her own death.

Chapter 7

Medical Uncertainty

Current television medical dramas such as ER, House, M.D., and Grey's Anatomy depict the brilliance of medicine and its doctors, but they also point out human flaws and the existence of medical uncertainties. The truth is that PICU doctors don't always know what is really going on inside a child's body. This chapter will tell you about an extreme example of that, a case in which we physicians never had much insight into what was happening, and how such total uncertainty affects the doctors as much as it does the child's family.

Eric was a seven-year-old boy who, like many small boys, loved dinosaurs. He had a huge plastic collection of them which he played with behind his house in the sand pile. One minute he was playing with his beloved dinosaurs; the next he was having a tonic seizure that landed him in the ER for several months. The following story explores different types and severities of seizures, the vast complexity of the human brain, the curse and blessing of powerful drugs, a mother and father's remarkable calm through their son's storm, and the absolute head-scratching vagueness that can surround certain illnesses and plague the PICU staff itself.

One Saturday while outside playing, Eric did not come in for lunch. His mother, busy all day, did not notice until early afternoon that she had not seen her son since he had taken his sack of dinosaurs out to the sand pile that morning. When she went out to look for him, she found him around the corner of the house beneath the swing set. He was lying on his side in the dirt. He did not respond at all when she called out to him, although he did move a bit when she shook him. He was breathing, but his breaths appeared to his mother to be abnormally shallow.

Eric's mother, like most parents in this situation, did not really know what to do. She had once taken a CPR class, but in that brief experience she had used a plastic mannequin to work on, not her own son. Still, she did what she recalled that she should do: she rolled him over, although this was difficult because his muscles were so stiff, checked for breathing and a pulse (both seemed alright), and called out for help to the neighbors. One of them came running to see what the problem was, then ran back inside to call 911. (Eric's story, like several others in this book, took place long before cellular telephones were everywhere.) The ambulance arrived in a few minutes, assessed the situation, and started an intravenous line. Eric was unchanged from the way his mother had found him; his muscles were still stiff, his jaw was clenched, and he did not open his eyes or respond when anyone spoke to him. However, he was breathing and the amount of oxygen in his blood was adequate.

Eric was still the same when the ambulance arrived at the emergency department. Alerted by radio, the nurses there waved the paramedics past all of the other patients in the waiting room to the place in the department reserved for critically ill patients. Such critical beds are fully stocked at all times with everything one would need to shock a heart back into life, secure an airway, crack open a chest, control massive bleeding, or, in Eric's case, stop a seizure. Because it was immediately clear to the doctor in the emergency department that Eric was having what is termed a tonic seizure. A typical generalized seizure causes rhythmic jerking of a child's arms and legs–called a tonic-clonic seizure. Some seizures, like Eric's, just cause the tonic, or stiffening part. After first making sure that Eric's breathing was alright, the doctor gave the child first one dose, then another, of lorazepam (the brand name is Ativan), a powerful anti-seizure medication. Eric's muscles relaxed; his seizure had stopped.

Eric had never had anything like this happen to him before. In fact, he had only been to the doctor for normal check-ups. So why did he have a seizure? Once it had stopped, the doctor ordered tests to see what had caused it. Had he fallen from the swing and hit his head? The quickest test to check for immediate, life-threatening things that might be happening inside the brain is a CT scan of the head. Eric had one, and it was normal; he had no brain swelling, brain tumors, structural malformations of his brain, or bleeding inside of or around his brain. His skull was not cracked or broken from hitting his head on something, such as might have happened after a fall. Even though Eric had no fever that would suggest the possibility of a brain infection, the doctor did a lumbar puncture, a spinal tap, to sample some of the fluid around Eric's brain to look for infection; his spinal fluid was normal.

By this time about two hours had gone by. Eric was still completely unconscious, but this could have been from the after-effects of the seizure (known as the post-ictal state) or from the drugs he got to stop the seizure, since lorazepam is a potent sedative by itself. He was still breathing satisfactorily, which meant that he had enough oxygen in his bloodstream. His heart rate and blood pressure were also satisfactory. Results from a few of the other tests that the doctor ordered began to drift back from the laboratory, but none of them gave us any clues. Eric had no abnormalities in his blood chemistries or his blood cell counts. When a child has an altered mental status, we always consider the possibility of some sort of toxic ingestion, but neither his blood nor his urine showed any evidence of a strange drug or toxin that could have done this.

The doctor was pondering what to do next when the nurse caring for Eric called from the child's bedside that the seizures had started again. Indeed, Eric was stiffening all of his muscles and his breathing was shallow and raspy from the clenching of his jaw. The doctor gave Eric another dose of lorazepam, then another before the seizure stopped and Eric relaxed. This time, however, either the seizure or the drug, or both in combination, caused Eric's breathing to slow down and then stop. The doctor had no choice but to intubate Eric's airway with a breathing tube. He also gave Eric a hefty "loading" dose of phenobarbital, a powerful anti-seizure medication. Although lorazepam works well for stopping seizures, we generally do not use repeated doses of that drug in this situation. Rather, if it looks as if a child will need ongoing seizure treatment, we switch to another drug. In the last few years there has been an explosion of new anti-seizure drugs for us to use, but phenobarbital was the standard for children when I cared for Eric. I wish that we had had then all of the anti-seizure drugs that we have available now. The doctor in the emergency department then called me about getting Eric a bed in the PICU.

Eric's situation when he arrived in the PICU was this: he was a previously healthy child who had experienced the sudden onset of severe seizures that rendered him unconscious; he remained unconscious to the extent that he could not breathe unassisted; and we did not know the cause of his seizures. In a nutshell, we had no idea what was going on. The medical description of his state is termed *status epilepticus*–constant or repetitive seizures coming one after another in rapid succession. I sat down with Eric's parents when they arrived in the PICU from the emergency department with their son and explained to them our ignorance, although for the moment I could at least say that his vital signs and blood oxygen status were satisfactory; that was something. While we tried to figure out what had happened to Eric, we would use the mechanical ventilator to breathe for him and anti-seizure medications to keep him from having any more convulsions. Everyone then settled in to wait out the night.

I have been in this situation many times before—a child has a severe seizure, gets drugs to stop the seizure, gets intubated, and ends up in the PICU on a ventilator. It is a very common PICU scenario, no matter what the underlying cause of the seizure. The situation usually resolves, or at least declares itself over the next twelve hours or so. What typically happens is that we wait for the post-ictal effects of the seizure and the sedating effects of the drugs used to stop the seizure to wear off, the child awakens and breathes, and we then take out the breathing tube. We next investigate what happened and take whatever steps we can to prevent the seizure from happening again. These measures may include starting the child on a regular daily dose of an anti-seizure medication or, if the child is already on one, increasing the dose. All of us expected that this series of events would happen with Eric.

The next morning, however, he did not awaken at all. He did not have any further episodes of muscle stiffening or anything else that might indicate a seizure, but he was still limp and showed no signs of breathing on his own. When I pinched him, he did not move. Even when his nurse stuck him with a needle to start a new intravenous line, he did not move. We had not given him any more drugs that would have sedated him, so it was clear that Eric was in a very deep coma.

About that time the technician who does the electroencephalo-grams (EEGs) arrived in the PICU. An EEG, often called a "brain wave test," is a measure of what the electrical activity is on the surface of the brain. Our brains actually run on electricity—current which is produced by the chemical reactions within the brain cells as they speak to one another. One way to think of our brain is that of a vast, incredibly com-plex and interconnected web of individual units in constant communi-cation with their neighbors. The patterns of these connections are laid down when we learn something. One could easily make an analogy between the brain and the worldwide web on the internet, with each user representing a brain cell, a neuron. Like computer uses, these neu-rons periodically log on and off, and they talk to one another with nerve impulses like internet users do as they travel to different websites with the click of a mouse. Also like the favorite websites of internet users, par-ticular neurons have preferred connections with other neurons. Finally, like the internet, the vast neuronal network that is our brain is diffuse; there are many pathways for signals to travel, and the minute-to-minute traffic flow of these signals is variable.

There are no unimportant areas in the brain. However, the neu-rons that control most of what the brain does are on the surface, the cortex. It is folded all over like a morel mushroom. The reason that the cortex has so many convoluted folds on the surface is to increase the total surface area of the brain, thereby allowing many more cells to be in the cortex than would be the case if the surface were smooth and flat. These folds are important, and you will meet a child in a later chapter who will show you why this is so. The cortex is where the action is.

Neurologists long ago mapped out which regions on the cortical surface of the brain control which activity. They generally did this by dis-covering particular patients who had discrete, identifiable defects of brain function, such as an inability to use a limb, a lack of sensation in a defined body part, or a specific problem with using speech and language. Neurologists could then tell, from where the patient's particular injury was, what function the injured area played in brain function. It turned out that many areas of the cortex are quite logically organized. For example, sensation and motor function for adjacent parts of the body lie adjacent to one another on the cortex. (One of the oddities of this spatial organization of the cortex is that the tongue and the thumb each have more cortical surface devoted to their function than do the arms and legs.)

The EEG test that Eric was having that morning measures the electrical activity of the brain cortex. It does this by means of a dense array of sensitive electrodes that the technician places on the patient's scalp in a defined pattern, covering the entire cortex from the forehead back to the nape of the neck and sideways down to the ears. When the EEG machine is turned on, each of these electrodes produces a wavy line on a graph that corresponds to the cortical electrical activity just below that sensing electrode. The wavy lines are displayed on a computer screen and the computer saves the information as it goes. The EEG machines we used back then traced the lines on sheets and sheets of paper, and by the time Eric left the PICU the paper tracings of his many EEGs made a stack to the ceiling.

Since the brain's neuronal network runs on electricity, we use the EEG electrodes to tell us what is going on in there. The EEG is a complicated and sophisticated test, mirroring the organ that it is testing. Although even a neurologist will tell you that interpreting EEGs is something of a black art, it is well worked out what the electrode tracing pattern when awake and asleep should look like in a normal brain. The key to that pattern is organization: the different regions of the cortex talk to one another in an organized way, with various neurons taking their proper turn to communicate with one another. A good way to think of a seizure is complete loss of that coordinated cooperation. In a generalized seizure such as Eric had, all (or nearly all) of the neurons of the cortex are firing off randomly and usually simultaneously. Chaos reigns, and when that happens most patients become unconscious because coordinated cortical activity is what keeps us awake and aware. (Some patients have partial seizures, ones which only involve a part of the cortex, and they typically stay conscious throughout the spell.)

Most of the time one can tell if a patient is having a generalized seizure, one involving the entire brain cortex. All of the chaotic firing off of neurons makes limbs shake and stiffen and eyes twitch; sometimes patients cry out involuntarily. Many adults with a chronic seizure problem sense it just before it starts, and parents of children with seizures can often tell when they are about to happen. Sometimes, though, it is difficult or even impossible to tell from looking at a patient that he or she is having a generalized seizure. They key is consciousness, and we always think of hidden seizures, so-called "electrical *status epilepticus*," in a child who is unconscious for no apparent reason, particularly if they have had seizures before.

Eric was just not waking up that morning, yet his seizures appeared to have stopped. The sedative effects from of the anti-seizure drugs that he had received the day before had long since worn off. Yet he was completely unresponsive and would not breathe without the mechanical ventilator. As the EEG technician placed the electrodes over Eric's scalp, I opened his eyelids to shine a light into them; the pupils of his eyes were getting bigger and smaller randomly and were not responding normally to the light. This was odd. Also odd was the faint flickering back and forth of his eyeballs—subtle movements that had not been there before. This made me suspicious that all was not well with Eric's brain cortex. The technician turned on the machine and started the paper running, and all of the tracing pens went crazy; it looked as if a bolt of lightning had struck the machine. Eric's seizures were back, or perhaps had never really stopped; he was in electrical *status epilepticus* in spite of all of the anti-seizure medications, and that was why he was still in a coma.

I am not a neurologist, but I did not need to be one in order for me to see the severe seizures on Eric's EEG tracing. I gave him a dose of lorazepam to stop the seizure; there was no change on the tracing. There was also no change after a second, then a third dose. I tried a different medication–still no improvement. Finally I gave him a large dose of thiopental, a powerful general anesthetic medication, and the pens tracing his brainwaves soon quit bouncing all over. His seizures had finally stopped. Thiopental stops seizures by stopping nearly everything happening in the cortex; it cools off the entire system by pulling the electrical plug. That is how all anesthetics work, how they put us to sleep if we need surgery and keep us asleep, unaware and feeling no pain, while the surgeon operates.

Thiopental does not last very long, typically five minutes or so. After I saw the results that the drug had on Eric's EEG, I left the machine running to see what would happen as the drug wore off. The EEG technician and I watched as the machine spit out the continuous tracings and the paper piled on the floor. It was soon clear that the transient cooling down of Eric's brain from the thiopental would not last. The wild swings of all the EEG channel electrodes recurred within three minutes. We would have to do something else.

I had already asked one of the pediatric neurologists to come and see Eric, and she happened to walk into the child's room as the thiopental wore off. She said that, as things stood, there appeared to be no way to control the seizures other than to give Eric deep anesthesia. This time we used a long-acting agent, pentobarbital, which induces a state of what we call "barbiturate coma." We have other choices available to us today in a situation such as Eric's, but at that time pentobarbital was the only drug to use. Eric needed a very large dose of it to stop his seizures again. Once they stopped, we began a steady infusion of pentobarbital through his intravenous line.

We use the EEG to guide the pentobarbital therapy, aiming to suppress the seizures without completely putting the brain to sleep. Looking at the EEG tracing, that translates to wiping out the wild seizure spikes but still preserving some background cortical activity. That is, we do not want a "flat line" on the tracing because that would indicate a brain that is completely shut down, or even dead. Pentobarbital has a very long half-life, meaning that it stays in the body a long time, because it is excreted quite slowly and tends to build up in the body's tissues, particularly the body fat. We do measure how much of it is in the blood and we have some guidelines to help us decide the dose to use, but the response of the patient's brain on the EEG is the best indication of how to use the drug. The only way to tell when and if the patient is better is to take away the pentobarbital and see if the seizures return; there is no real test for when to try to do that other than intuition and experience.

Pentobarbital puts patients into a very deep coma, and they need to remain on a mechanical ventilator for the entire time because they will not breathe or cough on their own. It is not a risk-free treatment. For one thing, keeping a child comatose on a breathing machine and other high-tech life support for weeks has risks. For example, the endotracheal tube can become dislodged, the child can get pneumonia from being on the ventilator for a long time, or the child can get blood infections from all of the intravenous lines. The chances on any particular day of getting these things are low, but over many days the risks are cumulatively high.

Pentobarbital itself has side-effects that can potentially cause harm. The most immediate of these is pentobarbital's effect on the cardiovascular system—the heart and blood vessels. The drug is a potent inhibitor of heart function. Nearly every child on the doses that Eric was receiving develops low blood pressure from decreased heart function. Most of the time we can counteract this by giving the patient another drug to make the heart beat more effectively, but sometimes this side-effect limits how much pentobarbital we can use. I started Eric on dopamine, a type of drug known as a vasopressor, which sufficiently improved his blood pressure so I that could use as much pentobarbital as I needed to block his seizures. His system needed a high dose of dopamine to accomplish this, however. Pentobarbital, over time, also tends to interfere with other body systems. For all of these reasons we try to get children off pentobarbital as soon as we can.

For nearly the entire next month we tried to do that, but each time we tried, we failed. Each time we took away the pentobarbital, his seizures quickly came back before enough of the pentobarbital had washed out of his system to even allow him to take a breath. Each time we had to restart the drug. It was frustrating and discouraging.

At this point some readers might be asking: what is wrong with having the seizures? If we are providing enough oxygen and nutrition to his body, what is the problem with that? Why could we not just let Eric continue to be in electrographic *status epilepticus*? As long as he was not jerking and twitching his muscles so that it interfered with the ventilator, why not just continue all of the high-tech life support until the process burned itself out, one way or another. After all, I have told you that pentobarbital is risky; perhaps the cure is worse than the disease.

In fact, brief seizures cause no damage to the brain at all, so long as the child continues to breathe and has enough oxygen in the bloodstream. Around five percent of all young toddlers will have at least one generalized seizure, typically when they have a high fever. This is because a rapid rise in body temperature is one of the things that can trigger something in the brain cortex to go awry and initiate the disorganized electrical neuronal discharges that begin a seizure. Seizures like this usually stop on their

own, although these so-called "febrile seizures" are a common reason for
toddlers to arrive in the emergency department in an ambulance. When
seizures happen, they look frightening to parents, who then call 911.

In contrast, seizures that go on and on for hours, and certainly for
days, do to damage the brain. A constant seizure for several weeks can severely
injure or even destroy the brain. To the neurons, having a very prolonged
seizure is like running a marathon. When all of those cells are maximally
excited and firing off their electrical impulses, they need energy to do
this—lots of energy. That means that the neurons need a huge amount of
the raw materials for that energy–sugar (glucose) and oxygen. After hours
and hours of firing, the body cannot provide the brain with enough of
either of those things and the neurons run out of reserves. When that happens, cells can die; the patient can die. This is why we could not allow
Eric's seizures to go on and on if we could find any way to stop them.

What was going on in Eric's brain? Why did he have a seizure in
the first place, one which came like a bolt from the blue? Once they
started, why were we powerless to stop them in any way besides keeping him in a deep coma? We had no idea what the answers to these questions were. This was not for lack of trying to find the answers, because
our PICU was located in a medical center world-renowned for its neurologists. By the time Eric's story was over, it seemed to me that every
brain expert in the institution had tried to help.

Eric's story is about the challenge of coping with medical uncertainty. Not knowing what is and is not likely to happen presents a huge
mental obstacle for parents and family members of children in the PICU
to overcome. You have not really met Eric's parents yet and read about
how they managed to do this, but they ultimately did so. Many outside
the world of the PICU do not realize that uncertainties and unknowns
bother physicians as well as families. For some physicians, the agonies of
confronting this obstacle drive them from even practicing medicine in
the PICU. Coping with the unknowable, particularly when lives hang in
the balance, is such a built-in part of PICU medicine that you should
read at least a little about this challenge from the physician's viewpoint.

After more than two decades doing what I do, I have found that
experienced pediatric intensivists share some personal attributes. PICU
practice does occasionally require quick and decisive thinking–perhaps

not as frequently as Hollywood script writers would make you believe, but it happens now and then, and often at unpredictable and inconvenient times. This is one field of medicine where minutes can matter, and the difference between correct and incorrect action can be the difference between life and death. This is the stuff of television and movies, and such moments are perhaps overemphasized in the eyes of the public. Yet it still is true that there are times when, if I make a mistake, a child may die. What most people do not realize is that such life and death crises are typically among the simplest things to manage. This is because the options in these situations are really quite limited and not much reasoning is required, just action.

In fact, a child who suddenly stops breathing and whose heart is not beating presents a straightforward problem with a standard approach to solving it. This is why good resuscitation skills can be taught to non-physicians, such as fire, police, and ambulance personnel, who have little or no understanding of the scientific basis for how the child's problem began in the first place. It does not matter; the initial course of action for a blue, limp child is the same. Some medical students and residents discover in the course of their training that, although they may be brilliant in their knowledge of medical science, they are not suited to critical care because they always want time to ponder things. Critical care is not a good career choice for such a person.

How a physician deals with the inherent uncertainty that surrounds cases such as Eric's is key to whether or not they will be effective practitioners in the PICU setting. You may recall from Chapter 4 the Latin saying in medicine, one taught to all medical students, that derives from the writings of classical physicians: *primum non nocere*, translated as "first, do no harm." The saying cautions us to insure, as much as we can, that our medical treatments themselves are not worse for the patient than the condition that we are treating. That was part of the challenge that Cody's parents faced in Chapter 4. You may also recall from that chapter a corollary to the admonition to do no harm, which is the venerable principle of medical practice that whatever problem exists may go away on its own without any treatment at all. Physicians use this therapeutic approach when we give the patient "a dose of tincture of time," doing nothing except waiting to see what happens. Both of these principles warn us to be wary of doing something just for the sake of activity alone.

On the other hand, the pediatric intensivist is occasionally faced with a deteriorating patient for whom "tincture of time" will clearly be followed by serious harm or even death. This situation may arise before the underlying cause of the child's problem is known. In such circumstances the intensivist must do what appears to be best based upon the best information available at that moment, even though subsequent information might show that it would have been better to do something else. You have read of a few situations like that in the previous chapters. But at least in those cases we had some idea of what was going on with the child. In contrast, we had no idea what was happening in Eric's brain or why. The stress of proceeding in a direction that later events show to have been incorrect makes some physicians, those who want more certainty before doing anything even if the patient is sinking in front of them, too uncomfortable. Such physicians are not suited by temperament to be intensivists; they may be brilliant at figuring out what is wrong with a patient, and excellent doctors on that account, but they should not be intensivists. Their psyche cannot tolerate chaos and uncertainty when there is a life at stake.

Eric's parents were actually coping with all of this uncertainty far better than most of his doctors were. At first, his mother's principal mental challenge was the fear that her self-perceived inattentiveness that morning had caused or at least contributed to his continuing seizure problems. All of the neurological experts assured her that this was not so. She agreed with their opinion because there was no evidence that Eric had suffered any injury from decreased breathing or lack of oxygen during that first seizure by the swing set. Once she was convinced that there was nothing different that she could have done to prevent the state that Eric was now in, she was willing to watch and wait to see what would happen. Her calm equanimity, which Eric's father shared, was an amazing thing to see.

I have told you about other patients for whom watchful waiting and supportive care were all that we could offer a child in the PICU, particularly Tiffany in the third chapter with her whooping cough. Likewise, with Ronnie's case in the second chapter, there were periods of time in which we did not know what was going on and what was likely to happen.

However, we ultimately figured out what was wrong with those children, so supporting the child on high-tech life support while their bodies healed was a positive and completely understandable part of our treatment plan for them. Eric was different; we really had no idea why his brain was acting that way, even though we tried for weeks to figure it out, and we had no idea at all if and when his seizures would go away.

Every pediatric intensivist has seen an occasional child with very prolonged seizures. In nearly all of these cases, however, extensive investigations ultimately show some sort of brain abnormality as a source for the problem. This is because most seizures begin at an abnormal spot on the child's brain cortex. These spots are places where the disorganized firing of a few neurons begins. Sometimes the chaotic firing of these renegade neurons spreads out from the abnormal spot out over the cortex until it involves the entire brain–a generalized seizure is the result. Neurologists often find evidence of these spots by looking at the EEG when the child is *not* having a seizure. This is because an EEG of a child during a generalized seizure may look like an unruly mess that is hard to sort out; after the seizure, the rest of the cortex goes back to normal, but the abnormal spot, the "epileptic focus," often leaves its fingerprints on the EEG for the neurologist to see.

Neurologists have other tests besides the EEG to help them find where in the cortex a seizure is coming from. The CT scan, for example, is very good for finding malformations in the brain's structure, such as missing or damaged parts, bleeding in or around the brain, and brain tumors. If any of these defects impinge on the cortex, they can cause seizures. Eric's brain CT was normal. Magnetic resonance imaging studies (MRI scans) reveal incredible details in brain structure and function, and are often very useful for finding the underlying problem in children like Eric. These scanners are now available at most hospitals, even smaller ones, although when I cared for Eric MRI machines were only found at larger centers. We had a machine, and Eric did have several MRIs of his brain; like the CT, all of them were normal.

Meanwhile, Eric was much the same. We were keeping him in a coma with the pentobarbital and, while on the drug, his seizures would stop. Every four or five days or so the neurologists would reduce the pentobarbital dose and see what happened; in every case the seizures came back quickly, long before Eric had even began to awaken at all. Each time that happened, we tried to use other anti-seizure medications instead of the pentobarbital, drugs which would not deeply sedate him, and each time only the deep barbiturate coma would control the seizures. We now have a wide array of new anti-seizure medications available for situations like this, but at that time our choices were much more limited. Even so, considering how severe Eric's seizure problem was, I doubt any of these new medicines would have helped even if we had them available then.

Throughout this entire time, now spanning nearly a month, we maintained Eric on full life support with a mechanical ventilator and tube feedings, although he had several problems. Once, he had pneumonia caused by the ventilator; once, he had an infection in his bladder and in his blood; and another time his intestines just quit working for several days and we had to use high-potency intravenous fluids to give him the nutrition that he needed. The pentobarbital continued to interfere with his heart function, and we needed to keep him on the dopamine to support his blood pressure. Fortunately, the dose of dopamine that we needed to do this was not a very high one. Sometimes children on long-term pentobarbital require high doses of several medications in order to keep their hearts working adequately.

After three weeks of this, we began to think about more extreme ways of controlling Eric's seizures. The most extreme of these is brain surgery. As I described before, generalized seizures in an otherwise normal child, one who does not have some underlying disease associated with seizures, nearly always begin at a discrete spot on the brain. If medications cannot suppress the abnormal neuronal firing at that spot, sometimes the only way to stop the seizures is to remove the spot–do brain surgery. Of course for this to work the neurosurgeon needs to know what spot to cut out. This is relatively easy if the EEG, MRI, CT, or all three in combination show where in the brain the trouble is. Usually the neurosurgeon, guided by an EEG-reading neurologist, first does an intricate mapping procedure of the entire brain cortex to identify precisely where to cut.

Such epilepsy surgery can work miracles. I have cared for children who have been having constant seizures for a very long time and who promptly woke up after the surgery and had no more seizures at all. It might seem as if removing part of a child's brain will handicap the child by leaving some neurological deficit behind, but in fact the child's brain had most likely not been using that abnormal part anyway, so removing it is not a problem. We asked a neurosurgeon to see Eric, thinking that perhaps brain surgery would help. The neurosurgeon spent hours poring over Eric's EEG with the neurologists, but they ultimately could find no part of the brain that was the source of the seizures.

There is a long list of inherited problems involving the brain and the various metabolic systems in the body that can first show themselves as prolonged seizures. We had experts in all of these diseases come and see Eric, and they ordered many, many specialized tests to look for these disorders. All of the tests were unhelpful. The doctors at one of the premier medical facilities for neurological disorders in the world had hit a wall; we had no idea what was wrong with Eric's brain.

Eric's parents had been amazingly tolerant of the doctors' ignorance throughout this entire time. To this day I do not know why that was so. I have spoken with the parents of thousands of PICU children over the years, and Eric's parents always remained for me enigmatic. Most parents would have been at their wits end after a month of this, by turns depressed, angry, and exhausted. Eric's parents seemed serenely confident that everything would ultimately work out or, if it did not, there was little that anyone could do about it. On several occasions I saw the astonishing spectacle of Eric's parents trying to cheer up and give encouragement to their child's doctors, rather than the other way around. It was the doctors who were having the most difficulty with how Eric's situation demonstrated how little we knew.

In the end, Eric's parents' serenity was justified. Finally, about the fifth time that we turned down the pentobarbital, the seizures did not return. The EEG still was quite abnormal; it showed how profoundly "cooled off" Eric's brain was, but fortunately it was not completely frozen. Eric had normal brain activity, although it was profoundly slowed down after a month of pentobarbital. Even though no other seizure medication besides pentobarbital had thus far worked to keep the seizures away, the neurologist began another drug, one which we could continue Eric on and which would not keep him in a coma.

Over the next several days Eric slowly awakened. He began to move his arms and legs purposefully in response to stimuli: when we pinched his arm, he moved it away, when his mother took his hand, he squeezed it. At last, after about a week, Eric began to take some breaths of his own, even though he remained intubated and on the ventilator. Soon after he would open his eyes and look at his mother and father when they spoke to him. Finally, he was awake enough to cough and gag when we passed a suction tube into his airway or tickled the back of his throat with a wooden stick. When he reached that level of conscious-ness, it was safe to try to extubate him and remove the ventilator. I did that one morning, and he breathed just fine on his own.

Even though he was off the ventilator, it took a long time–nearly another week–for Eric to be what most people would call awake. We expected this. For one thing, I have told you how pentobarbital stays in the body a very long time and how it distributes itself throughout all the tissues, not just the brain, and particularly builds up in the body fat. We were not putting any more of it into Eric's bloodstream, but the massive amount of the stuff that had gone into him over the preceding month needed to diffuse back out into his bloodstream so that his body could eliminate it from his system. This made him very, very groggy for a very long time. Ultimately, however, the drug was gone. Prolonged seizures themselves also usually leave a child with a profoundly depressed level of consciousness when they are gone, so the aftereffects of that needed to wear off as well.

For both of these reasons we did not expect Eric to return to his normal mental state for quite some time, maybe never. Since we never had a clear idea what was going on in Eric's brain before, we certainly could not make any predictions at all about what the state of his brain would be after his ordeal. And it had been an ordeal. Even though he had just been lying there in bed in a coma, his brain had been running a metabolic marathon. Only time would tell if his exhaustion left him damaged in some way.

As Eric was awakening, we continued to try to figure out what had happened to him and why. Now that the seizures were gone, we assumed that we at least would be able to see on his EEG where the spot was on his brain cortex that had set the whole thing off. His EEGs, however, did not help us. His brain waves were generally slow all over his cortex from the pentobarbital, but this slowly improved over time until they had returned to normal. By two weeks after stopping the drug, his EEG was normal—he no suspicious spot on his cortex that could have served as a seizure focus. The neurologist even tried various things to unmask a cortical focus. She did this cautiously, since she rightly feared that she might restart the whole firestorm in his brain if she stimulated it too much. But nothing that she did helped to show her why this had happened.

We also repeated Eric's MRI scan of his brain to see if his long ordeal had changed anything. We were particularly worried that, although he had not had any abnormalities in his brain at the beginning of his illness, the month of seizures and drugs might have left him with small areas that had been damaged from lack of nutrients or oxygen. But his MRI scan was still normal. On the one hand this was good, because we were looking for things that we hoped were not there. Yet on the other hand, his negative studies increased our frustration; after all of that, we *still* had no idea what had happened, or if it would happen again. Several of the brain experts were quite simply beside themselves with frustration, particularly over the issue of whether this would happen again to the child.

Eric, meanwhile, was making a slow but steady recovery. One of the fascinating aspects of neurology is that often just speaking with and examining the child is more enlightening than are all of the sophisticated tests. Neurology is preeminently the field of medicine in which a very careful physical examination of the patient is the most important test of all. And in spite of all of the normal scans of his head and his normal EEG, Eric's brain was clearly not quite yet right. We knew this because his neurological examination was not normal, at least not yet.

He was having difficulty in using language; sometimes he had trouble thinking of the words he needed to express what he was thinking, at other times he could think of the word but had trouble saying it. Both of these language problems are well known to neurologists, and they indicate some problem in the very discrete region of the cortex that controls language. This area is usually located near the left temporal lobe, which is on the side of the brain. It was as if his language center was intact, but just a bit out of practice after having been whacked by a combination of seizures and pentobarbital for a month. Fortunately for Eric, these problems resolved after several weeks of speech therapy. Using language, practicing it, made the problem go away.

Eric was also quite uncoordinated for several weeks after he left the PICU. He was wobbly when he walked, tended to fall over if asked to stand upright with his eyes closed, and could not write or draw well. His muscles were not weak, but he clearly had trouble using them normally. Coordination and balance are complicated neurological functions. The principal part of the brain that controls them is the cerebellum, located down low in the back of the skull. Anyone who has learned a fine motor skill through practice, particularly one that involves hand-eye coordination such as hitting a ball or shooting a basket, knows that constant practice improves performance. What is happening is that our neurons are learning new pathways to communicate with each other; once those pathways have been used many times, the act becomes much easier to perform. This was the case with Eric; with intensive physical therapy his problems resolved completely as his cerebellum and all his connecting neurons relearned what it had known before.

Two months after the paramedics brought Eric to the hospital, he walked out of the door to ride home with his parents. He had lost all memory for about a month of his life during the worst of his illness, but his mental functioning, including his personality, seemed to all who knew him to be entirely normal when he left the hospital. He still was receiving physical therapy and would continue to need it for another few months. I talked to his neurologist about two years later, and at that time Eric had not had any more seizures at all—not a single one. He was entirely himself again. The neurologist was too nervous to take him off his anti-seizure medication, but she planned to do that in another year or so if everything went well. She also had repeated his EEG and MRI scans about a year after his PICU stay, mainly because she just could not believe that she would not find *something* that would explain it all; the tests were normal.

Eric's life-threatening event came from nowhere and vanished as mysteriously as it had come. I suppose it is possible, with the many advances made in neuroscience knowledge during the last decade, that we would be able to figure it all out if he were to arrive in the PICU today. It is possible, but I do not think that would be the case. Eric's story represents the most extreme example I can recall of a situation in which we really had no idea what had happened. It seems entirely appropriate that his mysterious illness involved his brain, that organ which above all others makes us human.

CRUCIAL ADVICE FOR PARENTS

Despite the brilliance of modern medicine—its technologies and its doctors—there does remain the element of human flaws and medical uncertainty, a fact that parents must deal with during a crisis.

If your child suddenly experiences a seizure, it is vital to find out the events leading up to it; this can sometimes add to the correct diagnosis and treatment.

Pentobarbital, a powerful anti-seizure medication, is a miracle drug for epilepsy, but when used over time can interfere with other body systems.

One of the fascinating aspects of neurology is that often a doctor just speaking with and examining a child is more enlightening than all of the sophisticated tests.

Sometimes a life-threatening event comes from nowhere and vanishes just as mysteriously. In Eric's case, it was entirely appropriate that his sudden illness involved his brain, the organ that above all others makes us human.

Chapter 8

When Ethics
and Costs Collide

In this chapter I invite you to look beyond the particular stories of the next two children, compelling as they are, to understand the challenge of a more general problem: how the medical decisions that are made in the PICU affect not just the children in the hospital, but all of us. This is a perspective that makes many physicians uncomfortable because, when we adopt it, we are no longer simply physicians caring for individual patients. Rather, we become physicians caring for patients as an abstract aggregate of individuals—we move from patient care to Patient Care. Some physicians refuse to do this. As physicians, however, we must take some responsibility for the larger effects on society of what we do.

There are patients in the PICU who encompass all of our challenges—medical, social, economic, and ethical. Technology-dependent children, those who permanently require constant, high-tech life support equipment to survive, are such patients and, as such, are the focus of this complex chapter. Their situation puts a human face on abstract health policy debates. These children are not rare. There are many more of them living among us than most people realize, and their numbers are growing every year as the capabilities of our high-tech medical wonders grow.

Technology-dependent children's medical management is often difficult. They usually have complex medical problems involving many organs in their bodies, and complications of their many problems frequently land them in the PICU. In fact, there are days in many PICUs when children like these account for most of the children in the unit.

These PICU admissions are often caused by problems of one kind or another with the technology rather than the child's underlying disease process; machines break down, tracheostomies and gastrostomies need revision, pumps break, catheters in the blood stream clog or malfunction. We can fix the technological glitches. It is the other issues, the non-medical ones, that are the most troublesome. What doctors do every day, decisions we make one-by-one on individual patients, have an enormous cumulative effect on society.

In chapter four you read about Cody, whose parents met the challenge of deciding what was best for their child. They decided that they did not wish for him to join the growing ranks of technology-dependent children, using the four principles of medical ethics–beneficence, nonmaleficence, autonomy, and justice–to do so. Most of Cody's story concerned the first three of these principles, especially autonomy. I told you very little about the fourth principle, that of justice. The stories in this chapter speak directly to the ethical principle of justice, not simply for the two children in this chapter, but for all children in America. This chapter's stories personify a profound challenge facing all of us: how best to balance the needs and rights of individual patients against the just demands of our larger society, a society which already spends a larger proportion of our resources on health care than does any other nation on earth.

Ryan is now ten years old. He was first admitted to the PICU at the age of three with severe pneumonia. The reason for his pneumonia was clear to us at the time; like Cody in chapter four, Ryan also had weak muscles that made it difficult for him to cough and breathe normally. In fact, it turned out that Ryan has an inherited form of muscle weakness similar to Cody's problem–spinal muscular atrophy. Ryan, however, has a much milder form of the disease than did Cody. The underlying cause of the disorder is the same in both children; they both have a genetic defect that causes motor neurons to die. For children such as Ryan, however, the neuronal death is not so quick and so complete. We have no idea why this is so, why the cell death gallops along in one child and dawdles in another. Brain researchers believe that the gene that controls this process, although abnormal in both situations, is at least partly functional in children with milder disease. This allows Ryan to maintain his strength much longer than Cody, who had severe disease, could do.

Ryan recovered from his pneumonia, although he required several weeks on a mechanical ventilator and intravenous antibiotics to accomplish this. Ryan's parents were faced with a similar dilemma to that which confronted Cody's family, although there were important differences. By the time that Ryan was diagnosed with mild spinal muscular atrophy, he was a bright-eyed, interactive toddler. Most importantly, in Ryan's case the neurologists could not predict how fast his weakness would progress. It was even possible that, although he would not get stronger, his weakness might not progress much further at all. Considering all of this, Ryan's parents decided that they wished for their son to receive all of the high-tech life support machinery that he needed to stay alive. This was not a difficult decision for them, although they knew that it carried far-reaching implications that would be with them for the rest of their lives. I fully supported their decision, as I had that of Cody's parents.

Once his parents had decided what they wanted, the first thing that Ryan needed was a tracheostomy, a permanent artificial airway. This is how patients who will need a ventilator for months or years are connected to the machine. The children in previous chapters, who needed mechanical ventilators for only several weeks at most, had endotracheal tubes, devices which passed through their mouth or nose to connect them to the machine. These breathing tubes are only temporary. If a child will need a mechanical ventilator for a more prolonged period of time we cannot continue to use an endotracheal tube because there is too much tissue damage—a tracheostomy is needed.

A tracheostomy is a surgical procedure that requires the child to be asleep with an anesthetic. After the child is asleep, the surgeon first makes an opening in the middle of the child's neck, just below the larynx (voice box), and then inserts a stiff, curved plastic tube through the opening into the trachea. This device has a round hub on the outside to connect it to the ventilator tubing and its tip extends down into the trachea to a depth of several inches. The breaths from the ventilator then go through the tracheostomy tube down into the child's lungs. The tissues of the neck heal several weeks after the initial surgery. This leaves a permanent hole from the outside into the child's trachea, called a stoma. The plastic connection device remains loosely in the hole and is secured in place with cloth ties that run around the child's neck. It needs to be briefly removed and cleaned or changed to a new one every week or so.

Many children with a tracheostomy tube do not need the ventilator all of the time. Much depends upon why they needed the machinery in the first place. Ryan, for example, is strong enough that he only needs the help of the machine for about twelve hours per day, longer if he has had a tiring day. While off the machine, Ryan breathes on his own through the hole in the tracheostomy tube.

Tracheostomies sound simple. After all, they are really just a bit of plastic tube protruding from the front of the child's neck that connects to the breathing apparatus. They are not that simple in practice, however. For one thing, the opening needs to be sucked free of mucous with a mechanical device every few hours at least. Our lungs normally produce quite a bit of mucous which, in a child with a tracheostomy, needs to come out of the stoma or it will build up in the lung. We in the PICU get used to this procedure, as does the child, but to someone who has never seen it done, tracheostomy suctioning can look frightening. The suctioning itself, plus the strong cough that it often provokes in the child, can also look distasteful, even disgusting, to someone unfamiliar with it.

Speech presents another problem for children with a tracheostomy. We speak by moving our vocal cords back and forth as we are exhaling air coming out of our lungs. Our vocal cords vibrate, producing the sound of speech. These cords are located in our larynx, the cartilage box located at the top of our trachea, tucked just under our jawbone. Since the tracheostomy enters the child's airway below the vocal cords, the air coming up from the lungs does not pass through the vocal cords; it goes out the tracheostomy. If all of a child's exhaled breath does that, and no air goes up the "normal" way past the vocal cords, the child cannot speak, or indeed make any sound at all. We do have some kinds of tracheostomy tubes that allow a portion of exhaled air to travel up past the stoma to the vocal cords, thereby allowing some speech. In addition, many children learn to talk around the tracheostomy to some extent by forcing air up to their vocal cords. Even with these aids, communication is difficult for a child with a tracheostomy.

Ryan had once been able to crawl and even had begun to take some steps by himself, but by the time that he needed his tracheostomy he was too weak to walk. He could, however, sit upright by himself. By the time that he was four years old he was able to use a motorized electric wheelchair to help him get around. His arm and finger strength remain fairly good, at least so far, allowing him to pilot his chair around with controls located on the armrests of the chair. There is a platform on the bottom of the wheelchair that allows us to mount his ventilator on the chair so that he can be mobile and go to school, even during those times when he needs help with his breathing. There is also room under the chair for a suction machine and a battery to run everything.

Ryan is too weak to eat normally, particularly solid foods. He can swallow his own saliva sufficiently well that he is not drooling all of the time, but his occasional trouble handling his own oral secretions does cause him some embarrassment, more so than his tracheostomy does. He gets his nutrition through a feeding gastrostomy, a device that I alluded to in chapter four. A gastrostomy is a surgically-created hole between the stomach and the surface of the skin. Sometimes this can be done quite simply at a patient's bedside using local anesthesia and mild sedation, but children like Ryan usually require a more complicated procedure in addition to their gastrostomy; they often need an operation called a fundoplication. This procedure prevents liquids from moving backwards from the stomach up the child's esophagus (the swallowing tube) to the mouth. It thus prevents feedings from getting into the airway, which is a common problem in children with Ryan's sort of weakness unless they get the fundoplication.

Once the gastrostomy has healed, the hole from the skin to the child's stomach is about a quarter-inch in diameter. The hole is kept plugged with a capped valve mounted on a plastic button. This prevents any stomach juice from running out and it also serves as the connection device for using the gastrostomy. When it is time for the child to eat, one simply takes the cap off the valve, connects it via a plastic tube to a bag of liquid food, and lets the food run into the stomach by gravity. Most children Ryan's age get fed four to five times each day. There are liquid feeding preparations that contain all of the nutrients that Ryan needs to thrive. Any needed medicines also go into the gastrostomy as liquids.

In spite of all of his difficulties, Ryan is a delightful child and a joy to his family and wide circle of friends. He is talkative, having learned to speak around his tracheostomy with ease. He is an avid reader and master computer user, and is clearly someone with above-average mental abilities. The last time I saw him, now some years ago, he was involved in many activities at school. His weakness had progressed slightly, but he still was able to spend many hours each day off the ventilator. Whatever the costs of his medical care, and they are high, he is clearly a person who has and will contribute to his community.

Technology-dependent children and their families live very complicated lives. For example, a power failure is for most of us a minor inconvenience about how to keep the meat in our freezers from going bad; for a child on constant high-tech life support, such an event is a life-threatening emergency. All families like Ryan's need a plan about what to do when the power goes out. In addition, they need to have on hand reliable supplies of oxygen, spare tracheostomy and gastrostomy tubes, and all of the many odds and ends that their child's care requires. They need to have a plan for when the ventilator inevitably acts up or fails, an event which usually seems to happen in the middle of the night or on a weekend. Life for these families is complicated indeed, but it is astonishing how quickly most adapt to their child's needs and routines.

We have in our midst many persons like Ryan–individuals who have suffered damage to their nerves, muscles, or spinal cords such that they cannot walk on their own or breathe unassisted–but who still participate in our society and make contributions to it in spite of their disabilities. One well-known example of such a person was Christopher Reeve, the actor who suffered a severe spinal cord injury that left him completely paralyzed from the neck down. In spite of being totally dependent upon a tracheostomy, a ventilator, and a motorized chair such as Ryan's, Reeve became a highly active and visible proponent of expanded medical research on spinal cord injuries. He survived for over a decade following his original injury before finally succumbing to complications related to his medical condition. Another example is Stephen Hawking, whose situation I described in chapter four. In spite of his severe physical disability, Hawking continues not only to work as a physicist, but also to make major contributions to his field. Not very long ago all patients like these would have quickly died. We now have the technology not only to prolong their lives, but to allow them to live active and meaningful lives as well.

The mechanical marvels that keep Ryan alive are fairly recent innovations. Yet there actually have been a few technology-dependent patients around for half a century. The first glimmerings of what was to come with high-tech life support appeared sixty years ago during polio epidemics that regularly occurred before we had vaccines to prevent the disease. Polio virus is an intestinal virus in the same family as many common viruses that cause "stomach flu" and diarrhea in children. They are called the enteroviruses. Polio, however, has the unique propensity to attack and destroy the motor neurons in the nervous system. This leaves the victim paralyzed to a greater or lesser degree, depending upon how extensive is the nerve damage. A few unfortunate patients suffered total paralysis and could not breathe. The only way that they could survive was with a negative-pressure ventilator, the "iron lung."

The ventilators I have described to you up until now are all positive-pressure machines, meaning that they blow air down a tube into the patient to inflate the lungs. An iron lung works in the opposite fashion. The patient lies in a cylindrical, metal tank with only his or her head sticking out. A collar around the neck seals the device. When the air is pumped out of the tank, the negative pressure inside pulls the patient's chest wall outward; when the tank is pressurized again, the patient's chest sinks back down. Thus, he can breathe, although it means that he is imprisoned in the tank. Some patients survived for many, many years using an iron lung, although usually these were patients who were strong enough to spend several hours each day outside of the machine. When I was a medical student I cared for such a patient, a woman who had lived much of her adult life with the aid of an iron lung after having suffered an attack of paralytic polio twenty years previously.

Life-support technology has come a long way since the cumbersome iron lung. I do not question that we should provide patients such as Ryan the benefits of this technology, even though it is enormously expensive. I expect that most readers share my opinion. Children such as Ryan, however, represent the easy kinds of cases, those which embody no real ethical dilemmas. Many situations are much less clear. In fact, these murkier situations comprise the majority in my experience. To show you what I mean, I will next introduce you to a child whose story muddies the ethical waters significantly, and who challenges all of us with a very difficult decision.

Virginia is now seven years old. She was born with several severe congenital problems and has been admitted to the PICU many times for complications and surgeries related to these problems. Her bones and joints are crooked and she has needed several surgeries to fix that. Her urinary tract has a congenital abnormality that needed surgery. Her heart is abnormally formed and that needed to be fixed. All of these problems, however, are relatively trivial compared to the severe abnormalities of Virginia's brain.

Virginia has a malformation of her brain known as lissencephaly. In this condition a child's brain ceases to develop beyond the functional state present early in fetal life, and its surface is profoundly abnormal. As you read in the last chapter, the surface of a normal brain resembles that of a morel mushroom; it has a convoluted texture consisting of many folds, called gyri, and fissures between the folds, called sulci. The term lissencephaly is a combination of the French word for smooth and the Greek word for brain; it describes what the brain looks like in this condition—a smooth surface lacking the normal convolutions. The immediate cause of this severe malformation is a failure of the cells in the brain to sort themselves out properly and to migrate to their correct positions as the brain develops. The fundamental reason that the brain cells do not migrate properly in the first place is unknown, but whatever the reason, this failure to do so results in a profoundly damaged brain.

Lissencephaly is only a descriptive term. As is the case with many medical conditions, there is wide variability among children with the condition; in essence, some brains are smoother than others. Although all children with lissencephaly have significant problems with their nervous systems, the extent of the difficulties varies a great deal from child to child. Even so, all have profound mental retardation, most have problems with seizures, and many die within the first few years of life. Virginia's lissencephaly is of the most severe sort.

For Virginia, the situation is even worse because she has other problems beyond those with which she was born. To add to her many congenital medical disabilities, Virginia suffered an event that damaged her brain even further, beyond the damage already there from the lissencephaly. During one of her many seizures she stopped breathing, and her brain went without oxygen for a prolonged period of time. Her heart also stopped briefly. Many children would not have survived such an event, but Virginia did survive it, perhaps because her body was already so accustomed to such minimal brain function. So now, in addition to her severe lissencephaly, Virginia has another devastating brain condition, termed hypoxic-ischemic encephalopathy.

All of the organs in the body need a steady supply of oxygen. A few organs are especially dependent upon a constant flow of well-oxygenated blood, without which they suffer severe and irreparable harm within minutes. The brain is one such organ. Hypoxic-ischemic encephalopathy is the result of interruption of blood flow to parts or all of the brain for a long enough time period to kill brain cells. This is the condition that we worried about Eric having, the boy with the intractable seizures in the last chapter. Once brain cells die, they never come back. What happens to the patient next depends upon which brain cells die. As you also read in the last chapter, it is the surface of the brain, or the cortex, that regulates our higher mental functions, those things that make us fully aware. This includes our state of consciousness. These sensitive cortical cells particularly need a steady oxygen supply, and they are among the first to suffer damage when they do not get it. Virginia's brain cortex, already highly abnormal from her lissencephaly, was obliterated by the hypoxic-ischemic encephalopathy that followed her episode of not breathing during the seizure.

Deeper in the brain lies the brain stem, which regulates many unthinking reflexes such as coughing, gagging, and how the pupils of our eyes react to light. Even deeper in the brain lies the medulla, a structure which sits on top of our spinal cord as it enters the brain at the base of our skulls. The nerves in the medulla control the most primitive, or "vegetative" functions of our body, such as breathing, heartbeat, and digestion. Virginia suffered the most severe form of hypoxic-ischemic encephalopathy possible; portions of her medulla, plus a few parts just above it, are all that remain of her brain—the rest is dead.

Virginia's lissencephaly had always made it difficult to tell what her level of awareness was because her response to her surroundings was only minimal. The hundreds of brief seizures that she had every day made her state of consciousness even harder to discern. Below her cortex, however, Virginia's brainstem and medulla worked normally, so she breathed fine on her own. Her hypoxic–ischemic brain damage changed that. It destroyed key areas in her brain such that she no longer breathed reliably; she then needed a mechanical ventilator to breathe for her. Although Virginia is, in a sense, only barely alive, she is not brain dead. Her situation is what we term a persistent vegetative state, one in which she is totally unaware of her surroundings. Her vital organs, such as her heart, lungs, and digestive system work normally. She cannot eat, of course, and so she receives her nutrition through a gastrostomy. She cannot breathe, so she has a tracheostomy and a mechanical ventilator.

She has been in this state for years. Throughout that time her medical condition has generally been very stable. She no longer has any seizures because she no longer has any brain cortex alive enough to have a seizure. Still, she has suffered various complications of her life-support systems that are common among children like her. She has had several episodes of severe pneumonia that have required lengthy stays in the PICU to cure them. Any of these lung infections would probably have been fatal had Virginia's parents decided against asking us to treat them. If they had made such a decision, I and my colleagues would have supported such a choice. Virginia would not have experienced any physical suffering; her persistent vegetative state renders her completely unaware and unresponsive to the world around her. But her family wanted these infections treated, and her physicians honored their wishes and did so.

I have described Virginia's medical situation, and you can see that it is grim indeed. To make matters worse, her social situation is not a good one either. Her mother rarely visits her—perhaps once or twice a year—and when she does come she stays for only a few minutes. Virginia's father has not visited her in years. In fact, Virginia has never been home at all, in the sense of living with either or both of her parents. All of her many medical problems had kept her in the hospital since her birth, and once she suffered the hypoxic-ischemic event neither parent was able to care for the child at home. Between her visits to the PICU, Virginia actually lives with a foster family; neither parent has ever cared for the child on a day-to-day basis, and neither really knows what Virginia's life is like.

Both Virginia and Ryan are children who are permanently dependent upon technology to live. Both of these children are presently being maintained, at enormous cumulative expense, on artificial life support systems, machinery which ironically was devised to save lives, not prolong them indefinitely. This is the choice that their parents have made for them, and this choice has been honored by their physicians. Even though Virginia is in a medical foster care program, her parents retain the authority to make all decisions about their child's medical care.

Although these two children share a reliance on high-tech life support, they differ profoundly in crucial ways. Whereas Ryan is a totally aware, extremely functional child, Virginia is in a persistent vegetative state and she will never experience the world around her to any degree. Is it right to compare these children who differ in so many ways? I think that we should, and when we do so we must consider several crucial questions about them. Should the differences in their medical situations cause differences in the ethical imperatives that we apply to them; that is, are they equally deserving of this level of care? Does it matter that, whereas Ryan has thus far had excellent private health insurance, Virginia is on Medicaid? Does it matter that Virginia's parents are so removed from her daily life that the PICU staff sometimes cannot locate them for days at a time?

These are difficult, emotionally charged questions to ask, and part of the problem with discussing them calmly and openly is that the conversation is liable to slide quickly into generalizations. Sweeping generalizations are often facile, dogmatic, or both, and therefore ultimately unhelpful. When they appear, the conversation can easily degenerate into a figurative shouting match between opposing viewpoints. It is easy to have moral clarity about these issues when one does not deal regularly with their specific consequences. For those of us who do deal with these consequences, we ground any consideration of abstract issues in the particular events and mini-dramas that we live every day. This is how it should be; health care policy discussions should be rooted firmly in the reality of what is actually happening in individual cases like Virginia's and Ryan's. The world of the PICU can help us do that. It can function as a sort of demonstration laboratory for the key dilemmas facing health care policy decisions in America.

What we do in high-tech medicine seems all too often to be driven by what we *can* do, rather than what we *ought* to do. It is a fundamental economic truth that our society simply cannot afford to pay for all of the medical care that it is possible for us to provide—demand is limitless, resources are limited. Yet it is clearly unethical for physicians (or anyone) to decide about the appropriateness of life-sustaining treatment for a particular individual based upon the cost of that treatment. Money should never be used as an ethical criterion for deciding what to do with individual patients like Ryan and Virginia. But how are we to mediate between the rightful demands of society and those of the individuals who, collectively, comprise that society? Is it unethical for us to consider utilitarian principles, that is, of using our finite resources to provide the most good for the most persons? After all, last year my home state struggled to find funding to vaccinate all of the children in the state against terrible diseases like polio, and one year of Virginia's medical bills could have immunized most of them. Pediatric intensivists like me are sending more and more patients like Ryan and Virginia out from the PICU into the community. Is it right for us to do this without considering the larger consequences for our society?

Medical ethics concern a physician's duty to individual patients, not to an abstract collection of patients–the greater society. Indeed, the first three ethical precepts of beneficence, nonmaleficence, and autonomy essentially forbid physicians from using cost as a basis for determining the rightness of a course of action for an individual patient. Even the fourth principle, that of justice, admonishes us to treat every patient in the same fair way. However, the ethical principle of justice means more than this; it requires physicians, particularly those of us who practice in places like the PICU, to consider carefully how we spend America's increasingly limited medical resources. Justice for the individual patient means treating everyone the same; justice for all of America's patients means understanding that finite resources cannot satisfy infinite demands made for them.

In previous chapters we kept our considerations of medical ethics rooted in the solid ground of individual stories about particular children. That is life in the ethical trenches of medicine. We should do the same with medical economics. We can use the cost of Virginia's medical care as an example because her situation is typical for technology-dependent children. It is also typical in more ways than cost, as you will see. Bear in mind that these figures are costs as I write; as you read this, our inexorable medical inflation has undoubtedly pushed them higher. Another key point regarding these costs is that they reflect what Medicaid pays, and recall from chapter five that Medicaid never pays retail; it pays doctors and hospitals a deeply discounted price. Thus, high as they are, Virginia's medical bills are in fact artificially low.

The most costly part of Virginia's care is the nearly around-the-clock bedside nursing that she receives. Unlike Ryan, Virginia cannot breathe or cough at all on her own, so she is constantly on a mechanical ventilator. For this reason the skill level of her caregivers needs to be high, and all of them are registered nurses (R.N.). These nurses work for private home health care companies, all of which are for-profit enterprises. Owing to a combination of a nation-wide shortage of nurses and an increasing number of patients like Virginia in the population, there is often not enough capacity in such companies to provide all of the home nursing services that people want. This means that there is often a fairly long wait, sometimes six months or more, when we are tying to send home a PICU patient like Virginia. (While waiting, of course, such children are in a hospital, where the cost of their care is much, much higher.) Medicaid in Virginia's state will pay for her to receive twenty hours per day of skilled nursing care six days per week and twelve hours on one day of the week, at an hourly rate fixed by the state Medicaid agency. The remaining time, amounting to only thirty-six hours each week, is the responsibility of the child's family. The yearly bill for her nursing care is currently about $180,000.

Although high-tech equipment is expensive, it is the cost of skilled health care providers' time that makes up the largest portion of Virginia's annual medical bill. There are other personnel costs besides nursing bills associated with Virginia's care. She benefits from the skills of other health professionals who visit the child regularly in her foster home. In Virginia's state, Medicaid authorizes three visits per week each from both physical therapists and occupational therapists. Virginia receives both of these kinds of services. The physical therapists work with Virginia's muscles to prevent spasm and deformities, and the occupational therapists assist with her personal care and feedings. Medicaid pays about $19,000 each year for these services.

Virginia needs a mechanical ventilator. There are several varieties available for home use. They vary in how simple and how portable they are, with the smaller, more sophisticated types costing more. Ryan has a complicated and quite portable one because he often carries it around mounted on his chair. His ventilator also is capable of using several fairly sophisticated modes of ventilation, techniques that are particularly useful in weak, fully aware patients like Ryan. In contrast, Virginia's home ventilator is relatively unsophisticated because her persistent vegetative state means that her machine is constantly on and always functioning in the same way.

Even though Virginia's ventilator is a simple one, it is far from cheap. Patients like Virginia can pay for their ventilator in one of two ways: some patients purchase the ventilator outright, at a cost of about $10,000; others rent them on a monthly basis for about $1,600, which includes the oxygen needed to go into the machine. If the family (or their health insurer) buys the ventilator, however, there must be two machines available in case one fails, and that costs more money. Ventilators wear out with constant use, so renting them often makes more sense then buying them because the home care company providing the ventilator will repair or replace the machine as needed. Medicaid in Virginia's state prefers to buy the ventilator and contract for a spare machine as needed. Either way, the annual cost for mechanical ventilation at home is about $20,000.

Home high-tech life support has other costs from necessary additional equipment and supplies. Some of this equipment, such as the chairs fabricated specially for each patient, last for years, although they do require frequent maintenance and adjustment: these chairs cost around $7,000 each. There are also expensive modifications needed for the family car (more usually a van) to accommodate the loading and unloading of the chair: these costs are typically in the neighborhood of $10,000 or so. Patients like Virginia require a fair amount of expensive consumable medical supplies, such as suction catheters, plastic gloves, and equipment for her gastrostomy and tracheostomy. These usually are purchased through the home health care company, and are surprisingly expensive even when purchased in bulk by the caseload. Virginia uses about $12,000 per year in such supplies.

There are also costs for medications. Most children on home high-tech life support have complicated medical problems, things which often require that they take a long list of medications. In Virginia's case, the annual bill for all of her medicine is about $10,000. It would be much higher than that if she were still having seizures, since she was once taking three or four extremely expensive anti-seizure drugs.

Finally, there are professional fees to pay—the doctor bills. Besides her usual physician, Virginia regularly sees specialists in neurology (for her brain problem), pulmonology (for her ventilator issues), and surgery (for care of her gastrostomy and tracheostomy). Many of these periodic evaluations require expensive tests, such as x-rays and blood tests. This is particularly the case after Virginia returns to her foster home after one of her PICU stays. Since I do not care for her in that setting, I cannot be certain what the doctor bills are for her outpatient care. I estimate that, at a minimum, these bills total about $12,000 per year—some years more, some years less.

If we add up all of these amounts, we arrive at an annual basic cost for Virginia's care of about $275,000, over one-quarter million dollars. This sum, however, represents only the minimal beginning; the actual annual costs for her care are higher still. This is because patients like Virginia are extremely fragile in many ways. This is literally true for Virginia. Her bones have been thinned and weakened by years of disuse, in spite of the physical therapy that she receives, and she has suffered several fractures of her bones just from normal handling.

Virginia is fragile in other ways, too, particularly with regard to her ability to fight off infections. Patients like her typically have at least one serious infection per year that requires hospitalization. These infections often involve the skin, the lungs, or the kidneys. She and patients like her also often need to be admitted to the hospital for various problems relating to the gastrostomy or the tracheostomy. When Virginia is admitted to the hospital for any of these problems, she needs to come into the PICU because she is on a ventilator, thereby driving her bills even higher. All told, Virginia's hospitalizations for all of these reasons over the last several years have generally cost between $100,000 and $150,000 annually.

Considering everything, Virginia's care costs on average about $400,000 each year, and so far the total cost of her medical treatment has reached about $1,500,000. Who can pay these enormous sums? In Virginia's case, it is Medicaid, the taxpayers. But what about Ryan? His family has private health insurance, at least for now. In spite of that, virtually all children like Virginia and Ryan ultimately have their medical bills paid by various government programs, although the details are different with each child. These details are immensely complicated and how they work themselves out differs from state to state. In general, some states are far more willing than are others in how they use their Medicaid programs to support the medical costs of children like Virginia. Virginia's state is one of the less generous ones, although this fact has not really affected her life very much.

Recall from chapter five that Medicaid is a cooperative arrangement in which the federal and state governments share the costs, although the states themselves administer the program within certain federal guidelines. Medicaid was designed to pay for the health care of indigent children, pregnant women, and disabled adults. To qualify their children over the age of six for the program, a family's income must be at or below the federal poverty level; younger children and pregnant women are covered at a slightly higher income threshold. As long as Virginia stays on Medicaid, all of her medical bills, the entire $400,000 each year, will be paid by the government. There are no out-of-pocket expenses for her family because, as of this moment, Medicaid in Virginia's home state has no co-payment requirement for its participants.

If a family has health insurance of some sort, such as Ryan's family had the last time that I cared for him, their child's medical bills are generally paid by that insurance. His family would still be responsible, of course, for annual premiums and co-payments. Health insurance companies, however, have designed for themselves an exit strategy that protects them from years and years of enormous costs from patients like Ryan. All insurance policies have a lifetime cap on the total of benefits that can be paid for the care of an individual subscriber, typically set at several million dollars. This may seem like a lot of money. Yet Virginia has already incurred bills of this magnitude, and had she health insurance she would reach the ceiling on that policy within several years or less. There is no end in sight for Virginia's bills to Medicaid; the program has no cap for individual patients other than the theoretical limit of the global health care budget for the entire state. At times I wonder if the bills for patients like Virginia will, over the next decade or so, actually reach that level of magnitude.

For those families fortunate enough to have health insurance, what happens when costs of caring for their children reach the lifetime limit on the insurance policy? What will Ryan's family do then? It would be very difficult, if not impossible, for a family in that situation to get a new policy on their own, since insurance companies will usually deny any coverage of "pre-existing conditions." The ranks of the companies that provide unrestricted health care benefits to all of their employees' families are rapidly shrinking as premiums skyrocket. Without insurance, the annual health care costs of many thousands of dollars for children like Ryan would quickly exhaust the resources of most families. At that point the family could at least qualify for Medicaid, although this is small comfort to the financially-strapped family. This is not a mere supposition; I have seen such a double tragedy happen several times in my career, in which a child's medical condition leads to his family's financial ruin.

What often saves the day for the family, at least in Virginia's state and many others, is that the technology-dependent child qualifies for Medicaid by some other means than a simple calculation of family income. One mechanism by which children like Ryan can enroll in the Medicaid program is somewhat round-about, using a federal program administered by the Social Security Administration known as supplemental security income, or SSI. This program was designed to give cash support to disabled persons who cannot work. However, children can qualify for SSI if they meet the Social Security Administration's definition of disability. This definition is complicated, and the process of getting a patient like Ryan certified as disabled is protracted, complicated, and burdensome to families and physicians alike. There is also a financial means test for SSI, the total amount of which is fairly similar to that of Medicaid. Whereas the formula used to calculate a family's financial resources for Medicaid purposes is quite simple, the calculation for the federal SSI program is complicated in the extreme. There are many things that are added or subtracted to the final determination of the family's financial resources that Medicaid does not consider.

The result of this tangled process is that many technology-dependent children can qualify for SSI even though their families would not qualify for other forms of government aid. Why does this matter? It matters enormously because SSI qualification carries with it automatic qualification for Medicaid, and this Medicaid eligibility that derives from SSI is special in another way—it crosses state lines. That means that a family with a child like Ryan can move to another state and keep the Medicaid eligibility for their child.

Even if a family has too high an income to qualify for SSI, there are other ways for a child like Ryan and Virginia to receive Medicaid benefits. These programs vary a great deal from state to state, but in Virginia's state there is something generally known as a Medicaid waiver. Other states have similar programs. What this amounts to is that a child with huge ongoing and future medical needs like Ryan can be put on a waiting list to receive Medicaid benefits even though the child's family would not ordinarily qualify for Medicaid by income criteria. The waiting time on this list for Medicaid benefits varies for each child, but it is typically about two years in Ryan's state for children like him. Thus if a family with health insurance can get their child on this list, it is possible for the child to receive Medicaid before reaching the cap on their private insurance. This is what Ryan's family hopes will happen; if it does not, the cost of his care will bankrupt the family. Then, of course, they would qualify for Medicaid. It is indeed a complicated, labyrinthine system.

Figuring out how to negotiate through this labyrinth takes an expert, and every PICU has such experts. They are the PICU social workers, who are adept at guiding families and their children through this maze of program applications. The result in my experience is that virtually all of the children like Virginia and Ryan end up on Medicaid, and that the state and federal governments, the taxpayers, are therefore effectively the payers of last resort. This may be a good thing, it may be a bad thing; I make no judgment about that. But you should know that it is something that is happening across America. It means that the political debate about government involvement in high-tech medical care, about the concept often loosely termed "socialized medicine," is over as it concerns children dependent upon technology to live; we already have near-total government support of the costs of caring for such children.

The debate on who should pay for the care of technology-dependent children is over or, in fact, never took place, because the system we live under just evolved on its own. It was not ill-planned; it was never planned. It just happened. Moreover, although medical advances in critical care have steadily increased the number of technology-dependent children in our society, our capacity to care for them is static at best because most state Medicaid budgets, including that of Virginia's state, are severely constrained by the legal requirement that the state not run a deficit from year to year. I do not foresee that this situation will change anytime soon. This returns us to the challenge that is central to this chapter—the ethical principle of justice. With demand for services potentially limitless, how can we justly set limits and fairly decide what services society owes to each child? How can we look at children like Ryan and Virginia and say to them and their families: "Yes, you can have this ventilator but not that one, this corrective surgery but not that one, this therapy but not that one."

Any clear-eyed consideration of the challenge to us personified by technology-dependent children must move beyond slogans, posturing, and cant. This is not an easy thing to do. Some readers of this chapter, as they scan the passages describing Virginia's complicated and expensive problems and her vegetative state of existence, will make the argument that the doctors should "pull the plug" on her, that continuing to honor her mother's request to support the child is a waste of precious resources that could do much more good if spent in other ways. *It is not that simple, and I am not making that argument.*

Other readers will assert that both the principle of the sanctity of human life and that of respecting patient autonomy (that is, of following her mother's request) compel us to continue full high-tech medical support for Virginia. Still other readers might counter this argument with the claim that continuing to support Virginia in her current state is, in itself, disrespectful of the sanctity of human life because, although it supports her vital organs, such care inappropriately prolongs her natural life and almost turns her into a kind of object. Once again, *it is not that simple, and I am not making either of those arguments.* Sometimes I believe that the more that I care for technology-dependent children the less that I know about how to solve these intractable problems, problems which get more intractable with each advance in high-tech medicine.

What do I think should be done with patients like Ryan? I think that he deserves all of the high-tech support that we can give him. If we, as a society, decide that to do so is too expensive, then we must devise a fair and honest way to divide our limited resources among the many patients who need them. It would not be fair to continue as we do now, with high-tech life support being doled out as a sort of random lottery in which those who are familiar with the system can get ahead of those who are not. At present, money is given on a sort of "first come, first served basis," at least until it runs out.

What do I think should be done with patients like Virginia? I think that respect for her essential humanity means that she deserves to be kept comfortable and free of pain. I think that she should be supported with all available high-tech machinery for a length of time sufficient for us to be sure that she will not recover, recognizing that such a deliberate course could take several years for some patients like her. Beyond that, and in spite of her mother's wishes, I do not think that it is ethical to continue full high-tech medical support because it violates the ethical principle of justice. Yet we continue to do so. Why is this? It is because, in our current system, we have always done so, and I suspect that this will continue until the flow of money slows or stops.

As a practical matter, all of us in the PICU often do act in ways that effectively limit medical care for patients like Virginia. We do this by declining to provide further advanced therapies and technologies, even though families sometimes request them. For example, if Virginia's kidneys were to fail, I would not offer dialysis treatment. If she were to develop cancer, I would not offer chemotherapy. My reasons would emphatically not be economic; they would be ethical. My ethical justification is that these additional treatments and technologies are risky and painful and that their ultimate benefit for Virginia would be nil. To subject her to them would violate the ethical principle of beneficence at least, and possibly the principle of nonmaleficence. We do honor her mother's requests to provide antibiotic therapy for infections and to fix the minor mechanical problems that arise with Virginia's ventilator, tracheostomy, and gastrostomy. We do this because those treatments are fairly simple and low-risk and do not represent an incremental increase in the level of Virginia's care.

Children such as Virginia and Ryan are emblematic of both the promise and of the curse of PICU care; they represent situations in which technology originally designed with the simple goal of saving lives has been applied to prolonging lives indefinitely. This technology is enormously expensive and it is a simple fact that society cannot afford to pay for it for everyone who might want it. So which children should receive it, and for how long? Should we use total cost per patient as the limiting determinant, irrespective of the child's underlying medical situation? Or should we apply some sort of "quality of life" modifier that might distinguish between patients like Virginia and Ryan? The first approach would be easier and perhaps more democratic; the second approach, although more difficult to apply, would be more rational in many ways.

My point is this: these difficult decisions are not medical; they are political decisions about the kind of society in which we want to live. Physicians like me have opinions about how to meet these challenges and answer these questions, but our opinions are not a matter of medical training or expertise. At present we physicians are floundering as we grapple with what to do with patients like Ryan and Virginia. Yet we are aware of our ethical responsibility to treat all patients equally. Our problem, which we cannot solve ourselves, is how to accomplish that goal of justice and equal access to all of the wonders that high-tech medicine has to offer.

The answer is not simply to spend more money on high-tech heath care. Throwing more money at the problem would only postpone the day of reckoning because our capacity to do more and more in critical care will continue to increase until a new financial limit would be reached. This is why the PICU really is a demonstration laboratory for many key challenges and decisions about health care in America. The technology-dependent child puts a human face on the most fundamental of all of these questions: what measure of medical care, if any, is owed by America to each of its citizens? Patients like Ryan and Virginia demand that we decide.

CRITICAL ADVICE FOR PARENTS

Families of children on high-technology life support need a plan of action should they encounter a power outage in their homes. What could be a mere inconvenience to most families can translate into a life/death situation for those with disabled children on support systems. Back-up generators will temporarily supply power until it is permanently restored.

In addition to back-up electrical power, families should also have an extra supply of oxygen, tubes, and any other such equipment related to their children's care.

It is important to have some working knowledge of government funded medical programs. In the United States, for example, many technology-dependent children qualify for SSI—supplemental security income.

Every PICU in this country has social workers whose job it is to aid families through the maze of applying for such programs as SSI.

Be apprised of the key challenges and decisions regarding health care in America today. It can be summed up like this: What measure of medical care, if any, is owed by America to each of its citizens?

Chapter 9

Carrying On

The stories in the previous chapters ended when the children left the PICU. The reader knows little about what happened afterwards, and this omission leaves you with an incomplete picture of what the world of the PICU is like. Life goes on, and for some children their PICU experience is only the beginning of a long encounter with illness and doctors. These children may face months, years, or even a lifetime of challenges brought on by their initial critical illness.

If your child has been in the PICU, you may even find that these later challenges dwarf those that you faced when your child was critically ill. This chapter is about two children like that. It tells what can happen after a child has successfully run the PICU marathon, but for whom life will never again be the same.

One girl, a toddler, had a strep infection that resulted in numerous operations and nearly killed her. Her mother, being overly protective once her child was released from the hospital, found it very difficult to let her play among other children for fear of another infection and another near-death experience. Her fear for her child was all-encompassing and at times extreme, but life eventually did return to normal. The other child, a 16-year-old bright, athletic boy also had a group A strep diagnosis. His infection, which resulted in blood clots, was devastating and ultimately disfiguring. Yet, even as these cases illustrate, most of us have within us far more resilience and courage than we might believe.

Megan was an eighteen-month-old girl whose mother, Pam, took her to the pediatrician for one of the most common childhood ailments–diaper rash. The doctor diagnosed a minor skin infection and prescribed an antibiotic cream, telling Megan's mother to bring the child back if the rash did not improve over the next few days. Two days later it was no better, possibly even a little worse, so Pam brought Megan back to the doctor. The doctor noticed that the redness and skin irritation were indeed worse, although Megan still looked quite well–she was playful and had no fever. He prescribed an oral antibiotic to treat what was then a mild skin infection and told Pam to bring her daughter back to see him in two days.

The next day Megan's rash was worse, and instead of bringing the child back to the pediatrician, Pam brought her to the emergency department of the hospital. The doctor who examined Megan noted that the bright-red rash now covered most of the child's buttocks. The edge of the rash, where the redness stopped, had a discrete, sharp border. The doctor made a mark on Megan's skin with a pen to note the edge of the redness; when he checked again toward the end of Megan's stay in the emergency department several hours later, the edge had advanced half an inch. There was an area in the middle of the rash that was oozing a small amount of yellowish fluid from the skin. The doctor collected a drop of this on a cotton swab and sent it to the laboratory to see if any bacteria were there. This could show what was causing Megan's infection and would help determine which antibiotic was best to treat it.

It was clear to the emergency department doctor that Megan had a significant skin infection, termed cellulitis. Her infection had gotten worse in spite of treatment with an oral antibiotic that usually cures the problem. In spite of this, at that moment Megan did not look particularly ill; she had no fever, her white blood cell count, which is often high in acute infections, was normal, and she still was quite alert and active. Her only discomfort appeared to be mild pain around the rash. The doctor gave Megan a dose of an intravenous antibiotic and admitted her to the general pediatric ward for what he assumed would be at most a few days of intravenous antibiotics. Usually such skin infections melt away after a day or two of therapy with powerful antibiotics.

Megan got up to her room on the pediatric ward in the late afternoon. Within an hour she began having a fever and was becoming first irritable and then listless. The doctor on call that evening came to see her and noticed that the edge of the rash was now more than an inch beyond the pen mark defining where the border of the redness had been only a few hours before. The rash was also advancing around Megan's body to the lower part of her abdominal wall. Things were clearly getting more serious, and the doctor on the pediatric floor called me to ask if I thought that Megan should come into the PICU. Infections can move very quickly in children, and I agreed that bringing her to the PICU was a good idea, if only as a precaution. What concerned me the most was that the infection was progressing rapidly in spite of usually effective antibiotic therapy.

I examined Megan after she arrived in the PICU and noticed that the rash had worsened in other ways besides just spreading quickly across her buttocks, thighs, and abdomen; the character of the rash had also changed. Earlier that day, it had simply been an area of angry-looking, bright red skin. At that time there had been a few small places that were weeping drops of straw-colored fluid, but by the late evening there were many more of these. In addition, the entire area was becoming raised above the level of the surrounding skin, and the tissue felt quite firm when I pushed on it. This showed that Megan's skin and the regions beneath, the subcutaneous tissues, were becoming saturated with fluid oozing out of the cells. This fluid was likely the same fluid that had broken through to leak from her skin surface in a few spots.

By this time Megan had received multiple doses of several different intravenous antibiotics, and none of them had seemed to be helping at all. In situations like this we need to use more than just antibiotics; we need to do what we can to clean out the invading bacteria and the toxic substances that these bacteria are releasing into the surrounding tissues. These toxins actually dissolve away the supporting framework of the normal tissues. Megan had an infection caused by what the media have termed "flesh-eating bacteria." It is a potentially deadly infection.

After I had finished examining Megan and describing all of this to Pam, I called the pediatric surgeon to come and see Megan as soon as she could. The surgeon agreed that Megan needed to go to the operating room that night, where the surgeon would open up all of the child's inflamed tissues and remove as much pus and other infected material as possible. The pediatric surgeon also called one of her colleagues, a pediatric orthopedic (bone) surgeon, to come and help because orthopedists are particularly accustomed to operating on the subcutaneous and muscular regions that surround the leg bones, and at that point we did not know how deep down the infection went.

Megan went to the operating room just after midnight and was there most of the night. The surgeons found some dead tissue (we call it necrotic) and removed it. They opened up the rest of the affected area and washed everything out with bottles and bottles of irrigation fluid, aiming to flush out as much of the attacking bacteria and their toxins as possible. After the surgeons were finished, the anesthesiologist caring for Megan during the operation left her deeply sedated and intubated on the mechanical ventilator because all of us expected that Megan would get worse, possibly far worse, before she got better.

Soon after Megan returned to the PICU from the operating room, the microbiology laboratory called to tell us that they had identified the bacteria that was doing this to Megan—*Streptococcus pyogenes*, also known as group A strep. This is the same bacteria that causes simple, everyday strep throats. Megan had never had a sore throat, although her ten-year-old brother had had strep throats several times in the past. Some infection-causing bacteria are hard to treat because they have become resistant to so many of our antibiotics. Group A strep is not one of these; this micro-organism can be killed by a wide range of antibiotics. In fact, most of the antibiotics that Megan had been getting, even the oral one given to her at the very beginning of her illness, kill group A strep. Why then had Megan gotten so sick from this infection?

Throughout this book you have read of the uncertainties and unknowns in medicine, even high-tech medicine; we often just do not know why particular things happen to particular patients at particular times. This is a difficult thing for some parents to understand and accept, yet it is true. I do not know why Megan's simple diaper rash changed from mere irritation of her skin to a trivial skin infection to a seriously invasive infection affecting her entire body. I do know that by the time that she arrived in the PICU she had a life-threatening condition known as necrotizing fasciitis. This condition can be caused by several different kinds of bacteria, but group A strep is well-known to do it. It appears that some varieties of strep get their special ability to do this from a bit of genetic material, one passed around among bacteria, which allows them to make the flesh-eating toxins. Yet even if a particular strain of strep has this ability, it still must get access to the child's body. In Megan's case, the raw and irritated skin in her diaper area was how the strep got into her system.

Megan came back from the operating room on sedatives and pain killers, intubated and on the ventilator. Caring for her over the next several days was much like caring for several of the other critically ill children whom you have met in previous chapters. One of the recurring themes of this book is how high-tech life support systems in the PICU come to the aid of children with a wide variety of problems. In fact, there are days in the PICU when most of the children, even though they have problems ranging from car accidents to near-drowning, look superficially the same—deeply sedated and on ventilators, their beds surrounded by identical hissing, beeping machinery. As you have read, although we can help some of these children with specific treatments, others we can only support with the machinery until they heal themselves.

Megan's situation was one of those for which we do have specific treatments. We continued to give her intravenous antibiotics, both to kill the strep and to prevent living bacteria from releasing more toxin. This was not enough by itself, since her infection worsened even while she was receiving effective antibiotics. There are several reasons for this. One reason is that even antibiotic-killed bacteria remain in the tissues for a while, and the microscopic cellular walls of these dead bacteria can still do damage. Another reason is that the intravenous antibiotics do not penetrate the infected area very well because one of the effects of the bacteria is to shut off the normal blood supply from getting there.

A key part of Megan's treatment was for the surgeon to examine her frequently and continue to remove dead tissue and to wash the entire area out with fresh irrigation solution. The surgeon did this daily for several days. Each time Megan went to the operating room to have this done her tissues looked healthier and healthier—the infection was receding. It was fortunate that the surgeon did not have to remove very much tissue after Megan's first operation; necrotizing fasciitis can be a terribly disfiguring problem if the tissue damage is extensive. Some patients even lose an arm or a leg because the surgeon is forced to amputate a limb that has been completely destroyed by the infection.

I recall that altogether Megan made four trips to the operating room for "debridement," the technical term for cleaning away the dead tissue. Between trips the surgeon packed dressing gauze in her wounds to keep them dry and clean. After Megan's last session in the operating room, the surgeon was satisfied with how healthy all of the tissue looked and she closed up all of Megan's incisions. Meanwhile the antibiotics were doing their work by first halting the progression and then turning back the red margins of the infected areas. Soon after Megan's last debridement I turned off her sedatives, reduced the settings on her ventilator, and then pulled out her breathing tube. She would need another week or two for her incisions to heal, but Megan made a full recovery from her terrible infection.

Megan's PICU story might first appear to be an example of another happy PICU outcome—a cured child and a grateful family. Ultimately it was, but it was a long road to reach there for her family. Although Megan's physical scars were minimal, her mother, Pam, faced another ordeal after they had successfully finished the PICU marathon. Pam's second struggle is not an uncommon one; it was the struggle to allow Megan to be a normal child. If you have a child of your own in the PICU, do not be surprised if you find yourself in a situation like Pam's. You may find, as she did, the second struggle can be more difficult than the first.

Most readers with children will have encountered *Streptococcus pyogenes* before. After all, some children have strep throats many times each winter during their grade-school years. Even though Megan herself had never had a strep throat—they are distinctly uncommon among toddlers—her older brother had had several of these each winter. Pam had not thought anything of these since her son always got better with antibiotics. Pam's own mother, however, had said that the boy should have his tonsils taken out, since that was how a child with more than one or two strep infections was once treated. In fact, at one time doctors removed tonsils as a precautionary measure to prevent strep throats. If one child in a family was having them out, often the other children did as well. These days doctors are not so liberal in their recommendations for tonsillectomy, but you will still find much variability among doctors around the country regarding this issue.

Pam and her mother talked for months about the advisability of subjecting Megan's brother to a tonsillectomy. The family's pediatrician was strongly against the idea. He pointed out that there was no evidence at all that Megan had even gotten the strep from her brother. Even if she had, strep is so common among children that Megan would certainly be exposed constantly to the bacteria, particularly when she entered school. Finally, the evidence that taking tonsils out prevents further strep throat infections is itself flimsy, and the notion is a controversial one among physicians. Pam told me that what really frightened her was when the pediatrician told her that Megan undoubtedly would get future strep infections no matter what they did. Pam said that she would be terrified that each one might cause a recurrence of the fasciitis.

Under these circumstances, most parents naturally try to discover any way that they could to protect their child from the common, usually trivial bacteria. Were you Pam, you would too. It did not seem reasonable to Pam that Megan's pediatrician could tell her that Megan could not avoid getting any future strep infections, but yet not to worry about this. How could she not worry? Pam's own mother was of the opinion that most children should have their tonsils out anyway, just as was done in her own youth. After all, Pam's mother said that she had never even had a strep throat, a fact which she attributed to her lack of tonsils.

Pam called me to ask, as a sort of neutral party, what I would recommend. Although I agreed with her pediatrician, I encouraged Pam to get another opinion, because it is always a good idea to get as much information as possible about your child's condition. I suggested that she take Megan to see a specialist in pediatric infectious diseases to see what an expert thought was the best thing to do.

The infectious disease specialist was very understanding of Pam's psychic plight, but after he had listened to the entire story he told Pam about the latest research relating tonsillectomy to recurrent strep throats: in sum, this research had convinced him that taking tonsils out did not help prevent strep. Besides, the doctor pointed out that it did not seem fair to Megan's brother to take his tonsils out because his sister had suffered a serious strep infection. After all, if a tonsillectomy would help, would not it be better to do the operation on Megan? The doctor was

not really suggesting that course of action, but in fact Megan's grandmother had already made a few telephone calls to surgeons asking them
to do precisely that. All of them had been unwilling even to consider it
because Megan herself had never had a strep throat.

The doctor then asked Pam and her mother a few other questions
about Megan. He told them that he wanted to make sure there were no
abnormalities with Megan's immune system, that she did not have any
problem that would make it difficult for her to fight off infections. Pam
and her mother were not reassured by his questions and his conclusion
from their answers that Megan's immune system was fine. They were
alarmed, particularly because as far as they knew no one had considered
this possibility before (we had). Because of their concern, the doctor did
order some blood tests that check immune function, and Megan's
immunity was normal.

The infectious disease specialist also asked Pam a few more questions that are a routine part of such an evaluation. He asked about the
household arrangements, where they lived, whether they had any pets,
if Megan had traveled anywhere recently. These were innocent questions
that the doctor asked because he was thorough in his evaluations of
patients who came to see him for infectious disease problems, and travel
and animal exposure are often important issues in diagnosing communicable diseases. To Pam and her mother, however, the doctor's questions
opened yet another set of possibilities of where the strep might be lurking, waiting to pounce again on Megan. In fact, the family had a dog,
and the grandmother frequently nagged Pam about keeping the house
cleaner. These questions made Pam nervous, but parents should understand that doctors ask them to be thorough and to get all of the information; we are not necessarily implying anything in particular. But if you
wonder what the doctor is thinking, simply ask.

Pam returned from Megan's infectious disease evaluation as worried as ever about eradicating strep from Megan's environment. Neither
Pam nor her mother still believed that it might be a good idea to take
out everyone's tonsils. But what about the dog question? They had had
the animal for years, and he had always been healthy, but they took him
to the veterinarian to see if the dog carried strep. The veterinarian told
Pam that group A strep was not a problem with dogs, and that dogs did

not transmit the infection to humans. He was understanding of their situation, however, and offered to do a throat culture on the dog. It was negative.

Pam decided to purge Megan's home environment of any possible place for strep to hide. She scrubbed down every room in the house with disinfectant, after which she painted Megan's room with a fresh coat of paint. In spite of his clean bill of health from the veterinarian, the dog got a bath every few days.

None of these things—the dog, the painting, the cleaning—affected Megan. She continued to do her usual things and seemed to be her usual self. She was not sick in any way. The wounds from her surgeries healed completely, and they did not bother her at all. She had amazingly small scars from the incisions, considering how many times she had gone to the operating room. What did affect Megan was that Pam was terrified to let her daughter have any contact with other children, particularly children who had ever had a strep throat in the past. She took Megan out of the preschool program that the child had been attending before she got ill, and was afraid even to take Megan with her shopping.

Pam was not crazy. I understood her fears, as any parent would. Her child had nearly died from an unusual manifestation of a common childhood disease: how could anyone reassure her that this would never, ever happen again? It was certainly reasonable and logical for her to do whatever she could to protect Megan from ever experiencing that again. Pam knew, of course, that life goes on. But how could her life be the same after Megan's close brush with death? It seemed impossible for her to let Megan be a normal child and do normal childhood things, particularly those things that involved mixing with other children, any one of which might be carrying an infection that Pam knew too well could be deadly.

Pam's husband did wonder if his wife were not at least a little bit crazy. She made everyone in the household wash their hands over and over each day. She kept dispensers of disinfectant throughout the house until her husband began to complain that the place smelled like a hospital all of the time. Pam told me that her mental anguish during the year following Megan's PICU experience was worse than it had been during the crisis of her daughter's illness. Pam's husband and her mother, as well as Megan's doctor, urged her to restore a measure of normalcy to her life at least by going back to work, but Pam felt unable to do that because it would mean putting Megan back in preschool and daycare with other children.

Finally, after about a year of this, Pam gradually was able to relax her vigilance. It helped that Megan continued to be healthy and to give every sign of being a completely normal child. It also helped that Megan's brother did not himself have any more strep throats. Pam found that she did not feel such an obsessive need to keep the entire house spotless and the dog so abnormally clean. She put Megan back in preschool several days per week, and the child continued to thrive in every way.

Two years after Megan's illness, Pam went back to work at a new job. She told me that at first she found herself wondering frequently during the day about how Megan was doing at school, but ultimately was relieved to discover that she was able to concentrate on her work without worrying about it. The last time that I spoke with Pam was when she stopped by the PICU to bring pictures of Megan to show to everyone. The staff enjoyed looking at the pictures, as we always do, but we particularly enjoyed seeing that Pam was obviously pregnant. Three months later Megan had a new brother.

Megan's family faced the challenge of allowing their normal child to be a normal child after her experience in the PICU, and they ultimately met and overcame that challenge. If you find yourself in that situation, you may find, like Pam, that this is not an easy thing to do. Yet there is another, usually more difficult challenge that sometimes confronts children and their families as they begin their life after the PICU experience. This is when children leave the PICU not completely healed, carrying with them persistent, serious problems that may last a lifetime. When this happens, the child and the family must understand and accept the child's new situation. This usually requires that they change their expectations and dreams for the future.

Carl was sixteen years old when got the illness that landed him in the PICU. He was a junior in high school and, like most of the children whom you have met in this book, he had always been healthy in the past. He was in all respects an outstanding young man. He was one of the best students in his school. He was an outstanding athlete, holding varsity letters in several sports and acting as a leader on these teams. Beyond all of these talents, he was universally well-liked. Carl was the consummate triple-threat young man: brilliant student, gifted athlete, and all around nice guy. He was the sort of child most parents would want their own children to aspire becoming.

Carl was the youngest in a family with several other boys. His older brothers were also highly accomplished, having all gone to prestigious colleges and then on to prestigious graduate and professional schools. Among all of their boys, however, Carl's parents expected the most from Carl. His parents also had the financial resources to give Carl every advantage in life. Carl appeared so perfect that his entire existence seemed almost to be a parody dreamed up by a Hollywood script writer or romance novelist. Yet in spite of all of that, everyone whom I talked to about Carl would first tell me what a pleasant and unpretentious young man he was.

Carl went to a boarding school and lived in a dormitory with fifty or sixty other boys. One weekend afternoon Carl missed lunch in the dormitory dining room because he felt ill with some nausea. His roommates were out most of the afternoon, leaving Carl alone to nap in the room. When one of them returned to the room just before dinner, he found Carl to be still asleep. His roommate awakened Carl to ask how he felt; Carl seemed a bit dazed, and he complained of a headache. The roommate told Carl that he should go to see the school nurse, if only to get some medicine for the headache, and the two of them went to the school infirmary across campus. On the way there, Carl complained that he felt dizzy, and that walking made his headache worse.

The nurse at the infirmary took one look at Carl and realized that he was too ill to go back to his dormitory room. She put him in a bed and took his temperature: Carl had a fever of 104°. She called the doctor who was responsible for the infirmary and described to him what Carl looked like—fever, dazed and incoherent, and with the beginnings of a faint rash on his chest. The doctor knew from that information alone that Carl was probably seriously ill, and that the school infirmary was not equipped to handle the situation. He told the nurse to call an ambulance to come and get Carl and to bring him to the emergency department of the local hospital; the doctor would meet them there.

The ambulance arrived at the local hospital before the doctor got there. The nurse on duty was an experienced one, and like the infirmary nurse, she could tell immediately that Carl was sick and getting sicker. She placed an intravenous line in his hand and began to give him some fluids through it. Carl was by this time quite disoriented and was unable to take his shirt off when the nurse asked him to put on a hospital gown. She was not even sure that he understood what she was saying to him. As the nurse removed his shirt, she saw that the fine, red rash on his chest had spread to cover a much larger area of skin than the infirmary nurse had described; it was moving down his arms and over his abdomen. When she took his temperature, she found that his fever was now up to 105°.

More disturbing than the fever was Carl's blood pressure; it was dropping precipitously. The nurse responded by doing the standard thing in this situation: she tipped the litter that Carl was lying on so that his head was lower and his feet were higher, and she adjusted the intravenous line to run wide-open, pouring fluid into Carl as fast as it would go. She put an emergency call out to the doctor to come as quickly as he could, and meanwhile called the hospital operator to see if there were any other physicians who happened to be in the small hospital on that Sunday afternoon—none were.

The doctor arrived soon after, by which time Carl's blood pressure was a little better owing to the maneuvers that the nurse had done. Small hospitals often rely upon the experience and good judgment of seasoned nurses because there are many times when a doctor is not immediately available in the building. Nurses in places like that must be ready and able to assume several roles. This nurse was a good one. She had astutely recognized that Carl was going to need a lot of fluid to support his circulation, and by the time that the doctor arrived she had therefore placed another, bigger intravenous line in Carl's other arm and had hooked it to another bag of fluid, also running wide-open.

It only took the doctor a minute to realize what was wrong with Carl, and he called for more fluids, an infusion of dopamine (a hormone that supports blood pressure), and a large dose of an intravenous antibiotic. He also called for a helicopter to transport Carl to an intensive care unit, because without getting any further tests at all the doctor could tell that Carl was most likely critically ill with an often lethal blood infection—meningococcemia. Just before he gave Carl the antibiotic, the doctor took a sample of blood to confirm the diagnosis, but he had no doubt at all what the problem was, and he turned out to be correct. Carl had meningococcemia, an infection caused by one of the deadliest bacteria known—*Neisseria meningitidis*, or meningococcus.

The meningococcus bacteria's natural home is the back of the throat. It is often passed from person to person by respiratory droplets, the cloud of microscopic particles that surrounds us when we sneeze, but simply extended close contact—living in the same room with someone—can spread the bacteria from person to person. Meningococcus is not normally found in our throats. However, at any given time, several percent of normal adolescents and adults harbor the bacteria for days to weeks at a time.

When a person is exposed to the meningococcus, one of two things happen. By far the most common event is for the bacteria simply to live in the person's throat for a few weeks, causing no disease at all. When that happens, such persons are called meningococcal carriers. Even though they suffer no ill effects from the bacteria, they can pass it on to others, who may not be so lucky. The unlucky ones are the small number of persons in whom the meningococcus does not just innocently live for a time in their throats; in these persons the meningococcus invades the blood stream. Carl was among the unlucky ones. We do not know why the organism invades the systems of only a few patients who are exposed to it, rather than everybody. We do know, however, what havoc meningococcus can cause when it does invade.

Meningococcus shares several characteristics with group A streptococcus, the bacteria that infected Megan. Both of them are easily killed by a wide variety of antibiotics. Both of them do most of their damage by releasing various forms of toxins, substances which damage tissues in various ways. So even though the bacteria are dead—nearly all of the bacteria in Carl's body, for example, were killed by his first large dose of antibiotics—the effects of these toxins linger to devastate the body long after the bacteria are gone.

The strep that infected Megan did its damage by dissolving away normal tissues—the "flesh-eating" bacteria of media reports. Meningococcus works its harm another way. Meningococcal toxins activate an intricate cascade of natural cellular hormones, called cytokines, that affect nearly every organ in the body. Cytokines regulate many aspects of how the cells in our blood vessels work. They normally are released in small, controlled amounts. Fulminate meningococcemia, the term for severe infection with meningococcus, leads to a massive release of cytokines. The effect on the body is catastrophic, particularly for the heart, lungs, and kidneys. All of these organs can fail as a result.

Deadly as the cytokine effect is, meningococcal toxins cause their most devastating damage in the way that they abnormally activate the body's blood clotting system. The condition that results, termed disseminated intravascular coagulation (DIC), causes a shower of blood clots to form everywhere in the blood vessels. You may recall from chapter two how Ronnie nearly died from large clots in his leg veins that were shedding smaller pieces of clot to lodge in his lungs. That was dangerous, but at least only his lung was endangered and we could catch most of that shower of clots with the umbrella filter that we put in downstream from his abnormally clotted veins.

Meningococcal DIC is a much worse problem because clots are forming everywhere in the blood vessels, especially in the arteries. These clots close off arteries, either by forming on the spot or by having bits of already-formed clot break off and lodge downstream in some other place. Either way, the result is to choke off the oxygen that the tissues supplied by those arteries need to live. When that happens, the tissues die.

When Carl arrived in the PICU, we were primarily fighting the effects on his heart and blood pressure of the meningococcus-induced cytokine storm. That was why he needed the massive amount of intravenous fluids and the dopamine to support his heart. These cytokines also make the blood vessels in the lungs leak fluid, which makes the lungs stiff, and which leads to the severe lung problem such as Robert had in chapter one—lungs like a brick, stiff with fluid in the wrong places. Carl was soon on a mechanical ventilator like many of the other critically ill children whom you have met in this book.

We managed to maintain Carl's heart, lung, and kidney function using the same sorts of high-tech marvels that you have read about in previous chapters. Before it was over, Carl needed all of them: the high-frequency oscillator ventilator for his lungs, several kinds of medications and machines for his heart, and the dialysis machine for his kidneys. He survived, in spite of many large and small crises of the sort that you have also read about before. The challenge for Carl and his family was to cope

with the devastating effects of the DIC, the clotting off of arteries sup-
plying essential oxygen to body tissues. Even though we found ways to
get oxygen into his bloodstream with our ventilators, without the normal meshwork of arteries to carry that oxygen-containing blood to
Carl's organs and tissues, those tissues die.

Most of us who work in PICUs have cared for children like Carl,
children with severe DIC from meningococcemia. The effects of this can
be badly disfiguring, and this is what happened to Carl. He survived all
of the lung, heart, and kidney failure, but life would never be the same
again for this charismatic, handsome, and talented boy, one whom life
had dealt so many advantages.

Carl suffered recurrent clotting in many of the large vessels in his
body. This problem waxed and waned over his first few days in the
PICU, but most of the damage was done during the early days of his
illness. The first sign of trouble was when he began to have areas of
whitish discoloration at many places over his thighs, and then over random spots on his arms and buttocks. The smallest of these were the size
of a dime; the larger ones were four to five inches across. The borders
of these spots were irregular, but they sharply separated the normal
from the abnormal skin. A few of them, once they appeared, resolved
by first becoming bright read and then gradually looking like normal
skin again. Most of them, however, went from a whitish discoloration,
to gray, to black. They turned black because the tissue in the spot–the
skin and subcutaneous tissue–was dead.

Each of these spots indicated where a clot had blocked off the arte-
rial blood supply to a particular region. They are called infarcts, and most
of the small ones were caused by bits and pieces of a clot in a larger artery
breaking off and traveling downstream until a piece reached a spot where
the diameter of the artery was less than that of the clot. The size of the
infarct indicated how big and important the blood vessel was; small vessel
blockage caused a small infarct, larger vessels a larger infarct. The process
was largely random, although Carl did have more of them in the lower
part of his body than the upper part. The infarcts behave, and heal, as a
large ulcer would. This means that, after a week or two, the black, dead area
sloughs off, leaving behind a hole. The hole is more or less deep depending upon the extent of the infarct. We put various things on these holes to
help them heal, but the result is always a significant scar.

Hematologists and vascular (blood vessel) disease specialists have tried various things over the years to treat or even prevent infarcts from happening in patients with meningococcemia. The most logical way to attempt this is to treat the patient with a drug that prevents blood from clotting. The results, unfortunately, have not been good. This is probably because, although the blood in a patient with meningococcemia is clotting abnormally fast in some places, it is not clotting at all in other places, causing the patient to bleed. Thus clot-blocking or clot-busting agents have the potential to make the situation worse by inducing worse bleeding, and this has happened in some patients in whom they were tried. Both a hematologist and a vascular specialist were seeing Carl every day in the PICU and neither wanted to take the risk of this kind of therapy.

Carl's DIC soon became much worse. The first large clot happened in his leg. His nurse noticed that his foot became cool and she could not feel a good pulse on the top of his foot or behind his ankle bone. Over the next several hours, all of his lower leg turned a gray color, then a dark blue. When the vascular specialist checked for any flow through the major arteries in the lower leg, he found none. This was a catastrophe. Unless blood started flowing soon around the clot in that artery, Carl would lose the lower part of his leg–it would have to be amputated. Over the next several days Carl's leg became black just below the knee all of the way down to his foot. One afternoon several fingers on one of his hands lost their blood supply. Next, a large black area appeared on one of his buttocks. Last, and most horrible for Carl's mother to see, came an infarct involving half of his nose and a portion of his adjacent cheek.

By now a battery of surgical specialists–orthopedic surgeons, vascular surgeons, and plastic surgeons–were doing their best to preserve as much of the affected tissue areas that they could. In spite of their efforts, it was clear that the surgeons would soon need to remove some of this dead tissue. Small infarcted areas, such as were present on Carl's skin, generally do not cause the patient much trouble as they heal. These areas simply heal underneath the dead tissue and then gradually push up the scab until it sloughs off. This leaves a scar, but the tissue heals wherever the blood supply is good.

In contrast, larger areas of dead tissue can be dangerous to the patient because they may release substances into the child's bloodstream that activate those same cytokines that made Carl so sick during his first days in the PICU. In situations like that, the patient does not get better until the wounds are all cleaned. After struggling with this situation for several days, we told Carl's parents that the surgery needed to be done, and that Carl might die if we did not do it soon. They agreed, and that night the orthopedic surgeon amputated Carl's leg below the knee, as well as two fingers of his hand. The plastic surgeon then removed the dead tissue from Carl's face and buttock. Within hours of getting back to the PICU after surgery, Carl's heart, kidney, and lung function were already much better.

From that point on, Carl steadily improved. His lungs healed, I weaned him from the medications he had needed to support his heart, and his kidneys no longer needed help from the dialysis machine to do their job. About a week following his surgery I began to reduce his sedative and pain killer doses, and a few days after that Carl was awake enough to come off the ventilator. His meningococcemia was cured, and he had survived the experience; at least half of children do not, often dying within hours after arriving in the PICU. Now Carl and his family faced a new challenge—carrying on with their lives.

The first challenge was telling Carl what had happened to him. His parents wanted to be the ones to do this, although Carl's mother had told me many times during the preceding days that she dreaded this task more than anything else that she had faced. The morning that Carl came off the ventilator he was still quite groggy from hangover of all of the sedatives, and I was unsure if he would actually understand much of anything that we said to him. He had no idea where he was, what day it was, and could not even tell us what was the last thing he remembered. His spoke only phrases, and those did not make consistent sense. I told Carl's mother that I doubted that he would understand what she was telling him. Her sensible reply was that, if he did not understand, she would tell him again tomorrow; if he still did not understand, she would be there all day, every day, until he grasped what had happened. Her greatest fear was that he would suddenly recognize his injuries and that she would not be there to explain them and to comfort him.

Carl's mother was right; she knew that there are some kinds of healing that are best done by parents. Good doctors know this, too. If you ever find yourself in such a difficult situation as was Carl's mother, tell the doctors what you, as a parent, want help with and what you want to do yourself for your child. In my experience, parents nearly always know best about these things.

I do not know exactly what Carl's response was when he realized the truth. I was not then working in the PICU, having gone off duty for a week after I had extubated him from the ventilator. When I returned, Carl was fully alert and fully aware of the extent of his injuries. He seemed matter-of-fact about them. His biggest immediate fear was what his visitors would say, his school friends, when they came to see him in the hospital. None had yet done so because they were waiting for Carl's family to give permission. Several of Carl's older brothers had visited, but no one else had come yet.

There had been a flurry of anxiety at Carl's school once it was known what he had. This is often the case with meningococcal infections that occur in closed communities like boarding schools or army barracks, because secondary spread of the infection to other persons is possible. Most cases are sporadic, meaning that they are not linked to other cases, but meningococcus is well-known to cause small epidemics. There is a vaccine that can prevent most of these outbreaks, and everyone at Carl's school received a dose of this vaccine. It is also routine to give a short course of oral antibiotics to those who have been the most exposed to a person with meningococcus, typically the rest of the family. In Carl's case the school physician did this for his roommates. The idea behind this treatment is that a few of these contacts may be incubating the meningococcus in their throats, with the organism poised to invade. It has been shown that oral antibiotics reduce (but do not eliminate) the chances of this happening. Although there was understandably much concern at Carl's school, none of the other students got sick.

By this time Carl no longer needed the PICU because he was not critically ill, and he went to a hospital room out on the general ward. I no longer had daily contact with him and his family, but I did stop in to see him occasionally, and my colleagues let me know how he was doing. The rehabilitation specialists were working with his leg, and he was soon up and around on an artificial one. Carl was already collecting examples of athletes who competed successfully in a wide variety of sports in spite of being amputees. As a practical matter, it is much better for a person to have a below-the-knee amputation, such as Carl's was, than an above-the-knee one; the preservation of the knee joint adds greatly to what the person can do easily. It also helped that his missing fingers were from his left hand, and he was right-handed.

His principal ongoing medical issue was his face. Part of his nose was gone, and there was a deep crater in the tissue of his cheek. He also had a large area on his buttock that needed a skin graft to cover it, but of course it was Carl's face that was the most concerning to everyone. The plastic surgeon began to repair all of the damage a few weeks later, after the tissues had healed sufficiently. This process was a lengthy one, requiring several operations many months apart. After the first of these, Carl was able to go home, and I did not see him again for about a year.

Carl visited the PICU when he was in the hospital once more for what everyone hoped would be his last plastic surgical operation on his face. It was a trivial one compared to the major reconstructive work that he had already undergone. He came through the doors with his mother, walking with only the slightest of limps on his artificial lower leg. He had a small surgical dressing on his face, but I could see most of what the plastic surgeon had already done. Carl would always have several scars on his face, of course, and his nose would never look entirely like a normal nose. Even so, the results of his plastic surgery were impressive. I had seen his face right after his first surgery, and I had assumed that his face would always look severely disfigured in spite of whatever a plastic surgeon could do. Clearly I was wrong.

Carl was by then back in high school, just finishing his senior year. In spite of his illness, he had continued to be an outstanding student. Like his brothers before him, he would be going off to a prestigious college the next fall. I asked both Carl and his mother what the past year had been like for them. They stayed and talked about it for quite a while. Carl told me, not surprisingly, that he at first had a very difficult time adapting to his new exterior self. He did not mind so much the fake leg; he told me that, in the eyes of adolescent boys, it was sort of cool to have a "wooden leg," even though now we make them out of fiberglass. He was even playing tennis on the leg, although he knew that he would never be as agile on the court as he once had been. Regarding the fingers, Carl said that Jerry Garcia, guitarist for the Grateful Dead, was missing one and it seemed not to have affected him much.

The face was the most difficult thing. All of us are image-conscious, some of us very much so. But no one is more image-conscious than an adolescent. Carl told me that for a long time it had been difficult for him to look at himself in the mirror. Eventually, however, especially as he saw the progressive healing of the plastic surgery, he got used to how he looked. He told me that he knew that others were getting used to it as well. The best test was how strangers reacted. Most of us, when we are thrown next to someone with a disfigured face, such as on a bus, react in one of two ways: we may avert our eyes, avoiding any eye contact at all with the person; alternatively, we do the opposite and end up staring at the person. It is nearly impossible for most of us simply to notice the disfigurement, but then to regard the person as we would anyone else. Carl said that his face had made it to the point to where he was "merely ugly," and he said that many persons were more naturally ugly than he now was. When all of the surgery was done, Carl's stated goal was to move from being "sort of ugly" to the ranks of the "not good looking," a category that, after all, includes very many of us.

Both Carl and Megan survived their illnesses and, when last I saw them, were coping well with the after-effects of their PICU ordeal. Not all children and their families achieve this, but in my experience most do. Their stories teach us that, in spite of our fears and anxieties, most of us have deeper wells of strength and courage than we think, and that hope for a brighter future after serious illness is, for most of us, more than a hope—it is an entirely reasonable expectation.

CRITICAL ADVICE FOR PARENTS

The more you know about your child's problem, the better PICU parent you will be. There are many ways to get this knowledge, including asking questions, reading books and searching the internet. If necessary, ask your doctor about where to look.

Even with accurate knowledge, you may have irrational fears about what will happen to your child; this is normal, and does not make you a bad parent. Discuss these fears with your doctor.

Children are highly adaptable and will adjust to injury or disability if we are honest and straightforward with the information we present them.

Life goes on—no matter what happens to your child in the PICU, most families are extraordinarily resilient, and yours can be, too.

Chapter 10

Miracles Do Happen

This final chapter is about miracles, and is a fitting end to our collection of parables. You read in chapter six how Shelly's father waited patiently and hopefully for a miracle to save his daughter's life, and how he decided that one would not come. Many parents find themselves facing a similar challenge—hoping and praying that the doctors are wrong and that their child will recover from injury or disease. If you find yourself in such a situation know that, in fact, sometimes the doctors are wrong and a child whose situation is medically hopeless survives against all odds. Even more astonishing, once in a great while such a child not only survives, but goes on to make a complete recovery after being on the edge of death.

I have cared for several memorable children like that over the years. They are the children who have taught me never to tell a family that I know for certain what will happen—I don't. This chapter tells the story of a child like that, a 17-year-old girl who had bleeding on the brain. Most doctors in the PICU didn't think she would live another day. Yet she recovered, suddenly and some would say miraculously, with her medically-trained mother at her side.

Carrie was an only child who lived with her mother, Joan. She was an extremely intelligent girl, a brilliant student in fact, who was making plans to attend one of the several prestigious colleges and universities that had offered her admission for the next fall's freshman class. Carrie's mother was also quite intelligent, and was a highly trained professional woman. She had a wide circle of friends, many of whom were also professionals of various sorts, particularly doctors and lawyers. This sort of social background for a child in the PICU can make the staff nervous. All of us strive to treat every child the same, but it can be disconcerting to have physician colleagues and attorneys who practice personal injury law visiting the PICU.

Carrie came into the PICU one night. She had felt fine all day and had not been recently ill in any way. She and her mother were getting ready to eat dinner. Her mother was still in the kitchen and Carrie was carrying the food into the dining room, when her mother heard a crash. When her mother ran into the dining room, she found Carrie lying on the floor in a pile of broken dishes. The child was twitching her arms and legs in what her mother knew to be a generalized seizure of the kind we term a tonic-clonic seizure. This was a different kind of seizure than Eric, the boy in chapter seven, had experienced; he had been rigidly stiff all over, a tonic seizure. The implications of Carrie's seizure, however, were the same as Eric's had been. Both meant that the brain cortex was experiencing a storm of uncontrolled electrical nerve discharges sufficient to make the child unconscious.

Unlike Eric, Carrie awakened quickly from her seizure. It lasted only about two minutes or so altogether. She appeared to have hit her head on the table as she collapsed on the floor because there was a cut above one of her eyes and some blood on the edge of the table. Joan had arrived in the room just seconds after the seizure had started and she had noticed that, although Carrie's lips were a bit dusky, the child was breathing. As her mother moved to turn Carrie on her side and check to make sure that there was nothing in her airway that might block it, the seizure stopped. By the time the ambulance arrived at the house ten minutes later, Carrie was moaning but was also responding to commands such as "squeeze my hand." When the ambulance reached the hospital another ten minutes after that Carrie was groggy, but awake, and nearly back to her usual self.

The doctor in the emergency department, as had been the case with Eric, did some tests to try to determine what the cause of Carrie's seizure was. He was particularly interested in trying to determine which of these two scenarios had happened: had Carrie stumbled, fallen, hit her head, and then had a seizure (a so-called "post-traumatic seizure"); or had she first experienced her seizure while standing up, collapsed unconsciousness as a result of the seizure, and then hit her head on the way down to the floor while still convulsing. The distinction between these two possibilities was important. Carrie herself was not much help to the doctor because she could not remember what had happened. In fact, she could not remember even having gone into the dining room.

Memory loss after a seizure is common. As you read in chapter seven, by the time that Eric came around from his very prolonged seizures he had lost over a month of his past life. Foggy memory after a blow on the head is also common, when it is called a concussion. This is a word you will hear tossed around frequently in conversation, but when a neurologist or neurosurgeon uses the word concussion, it means a brief interruption in neurological function, usually memory, but other things such as double-vision can happen. Mild concussions typically cause a person to lose memory of everything that occurred for several minutes before the blow to the head. That is why you will see a trainer on the sidelines of a football game asking a player hit on the head what the last thing is that they remember; the trainer is trying to decide if the player has had a concussion. The cut on Carrie's scalp showed that she had hit her head quite hard, certainly hard enough to concuss her brain. Carrie was by this time alert and cooperative as she was talking to the doctor, but she did complain of a dull headache and some nausea. The doctor in the emergency department sent Carrie down the hall for a CT scan of her head. This would not tell him much about the seizure, but it would tell him if she had cracked her skull or bruised her brain.

The CT scan showed the doctor what was wrong, at least at that point: Carrie had suffered bleeding inside of her brain, termed an intracerebral hemorrhage. The area affected by the bleeding was small. It was in the left temporal lobe of the brain, around a region of the cortex that controls how the brain understands and uses speech. At that moment, however, Carrie's speech was normal. The CT scan also showed that there was quite a bit of tissue swelling around where she had cut her scalp. There was no skull fracture, however. Most importantly, her brain itself was not swollen. She had a collection of blood about the size of a marble in the middle of her temporal lobe, but the region around this was not affected. The doctor in the emergency department still did not know what had really happened, but it seemed to him most likely that Carrie had experienced the bleed, which had caused a seizure, which had made her fall, which had caused her to strike her head on the table.

Neurosurgeons are the experts at managing this kind of problem, and one evaluated Carrie in the emergency department. He talked to Carrie and her mother, found her neurological examination to be normal, and reviewed the CT scan of her head. The thing to do at that point was to admit Carrie to the PICU for close observation, in case she had further bleeding or more seizures, and plan some further tests to help him figure out why she had suffered the apparently sudden and spontaneous bleeding in her brain. By the time that Carrie got up to the PICU it was the middle of the night. She felt well except for some pain over her newly stitched-up cut. Her nausea was gone and she asked me if it was too late to get her some dinner. I took this as a good sign that she was better.

I examined Carrie and found that nothing had changed from her normal neurological examination in the emergency department. At that hour the nurses only had some crackers to offer Carrie, but her mother went out and got her a pizza. Joan helped her eat it and then stayed with her daughter all night, dozing in a chair beside the bed. I ordered some tests for the morning that would start our investigation to figure out why she had experienced the bleeding in her brain. Carrie fell asleep about two o'clock in the morning. While she was asleep, the PICU nurses continued to check on her every hour to make sure that her neurological situation had not changed. After all, that was why she was in the PICU– so that we could watch her closely.

Our biggest fear was that Carrie would bleed again from the same spot in her brain. When this happens, the second bleeding episode can be much worse than the first and the child may suffer severe brain injury or even die. One consideration is if the child has an inherited bleeding problem, a tendency to bleed because of some defect in the blood clotting mechanism. There are many kinds of these disorders–derangements caused by too much or too little blood clotting–and more of them are being discovered all of the time. Carrie's story took place two decades ago, and at that time our ability to detect bleeding and clotting problems was much more limited than it is now. Still, I knew from the tests that had been done in the emergency department that Carrie did not have a major bleeding disease. This was important to know, because if she had such a problem she likely would have needed treatment of some kind right away.

I walked back into the PICU the next morning around seven o'clock. Carrie's nurse had last checked on her at six, and, although the child was still asleep, she aroused easily and answered a few standard questions such as: "Where are you?" The pupils of her eyes were also normal, meaning that they were equal in diameter and they constricted normally when the nurse shined a penlight into them. Joan was still sleeping in the chair.

As I sat down at the nursing station desk, Joan came out of the child's room to find a nurse. The nursing shifts were just changing, and Carrie's night nurse was briefing her day nurse on the child's situation. Joan told them both that her daughter seemed to be "sleeping funny" and would not respond when her mother spoke to her. All three of them then went back into Carrie's room to check on the child. I could hear them speaking to her in a loud voice: "Carrie, open your eyes"; "Carrie, squeeze my hand." Then one of the nurses stuck her head out of the room and waved at me to come quickly, while the other ran for the "crash cart," the tall wheeled cart that you will see parked at the ready in every PICU. It contains everything one needs–tubes, lines, needles, drugs, defibrillator (electrical heart shocker)–to secure an airway or restart a stopped heart.

When I got to Carrie's bedside, I could easily see that something was terribly wrong with the child. Carrie was lying on her back, apparently staring up at the ceiling. She did not move when I called out to her or when I shook or pinched her arm. She was breathing quite deeply, even abnormally so, and her heart rate, which had been in the normal range only an hour before, was steadily slowing minute by minute. What disturbed me the most was what I saw when I looked into her eyes with a penlight; whereas her right pupil was intermediate in size, her left pupil was huge–widely dilated–and did not constrict as it should have when I shined the light into it.

Every physician caring for the critically ill knows what the combination of unresponsiveness, decreased breathing, a slowing heart rate, and a "blown pupil" means: Carrie was experiencing the early stages of brain herniation. The temporal lobe of her brain was pushing down on her brain stem, squeezing the vital control centers that keep us alive. You may recall reading about this feared turn of events in the first chapter, when Robert's brain began to swell. Complete brain herniation is always fatal. Fortunately for Robert, he never had that. I did not know what catastrophe had happened inside Carrie's head, but I assumed that she had suddenly experienced a large bleed in the same spot in her brain where she had bled the previous evening–the left temporal lobe. At that moment it did not really matter what had happened to start the process, because if we could not reverse the herniation Carrie would be dead in minutes.

Intensive care therapies have advanced in many ways since then, but management of Carrie's particular situation remains essentially the same today, which is to try to reduce the brain swelling while supporting the child's heart and lung function. In spite of all of the sophisticated high-tech tools that we have in the PICU, our ability to control brain swelling remains relatively low-tech. It is a paradox; we now have wonderful technology to measure the swelling within the brain itself, to tell us exactly how bad it is minute to minute, but we have only limited ways of improving the situation. At that moment there were only a few things that I could try, hoping that they would work.

The first thing to do was to give Carrie a large intravenous dose of a general anesthetic. Doses like these put people to sleep nearly instantly. Even though she could not be any deeper asleep, being comatose already, the anesthetic would drop the pressure building up inside of her brain. The drug does not do this for very long, but it is one of the things that we can do to interrupt or even reverse the herniation until we could at least figure out what was going on. The anesthetic would abolish her own breathing reflex, meaning that I would need to take over breathing for her with an endotracheal tube and a mechanical ventilator. I needed to do this anyway, however, since she, like Robert in chapter one, was too comatose to breathe reliably on her own.

The endotracheal tube would also allow me to use the second of the tools that I had to drop the pressure inside her brain–hyperventilation. Used judiciously, giving Carrie larger and more frequent breaths than normal on the ventilator would lower the pressure inside her brain, at least for a few hours or so. The third tool that I had was to give her mannitol, a drug which can lower the brain pressure, although it takes several hours to work. I used all three of these approaches. Within about five minutes, Carrie's pupils were again equal, meaning that her impending brain herniation had reversed itself, at least for the moment.

Why would a previously normal girl like Carrie suddenly have bleeding in her brain? We already knew that it was not because she had a problem with blood clotting, an innate bleeding tendency. In adults, high blood pressure is a common cause of bleeding in the brain, when it is called a hemorrhagic stroke. But Carrie's blood pressure was normal. Sometimes people who have a generalized inflammation throughout their bodies, such as the lupus that Esperanza had in chapter five, experience bleeding in their brains. These three possibilities—bleeding tendencies, high blood pressure, and inflammatory diseases (so-called "vasculitis")—are systemic problems, meaning that they affect the entire body. There are also problems localized to a single spot in the brain, certain kinds of brain malformations, which can cause bleeding. In fact, discrete malformations of the blood vessels in the brain are the most common cause in children of intracerebral hemorrhage. Perhaps Carrie had one of these.

There are several kinds of such blood vessel malformations. One type is called an intracerebral aneurysm. An aneurysm is a weak spot in the wall of an artery that causes a sack filled with blood to protrude from it, sort of like a weak spot on an old-time tire inner-tube. These represent ticking time bombs for the brain; if they get big enough, they burst and can cause catastrophic bleeding. Until that happens, they cause no symptoms at all to tell the person that the aneurysm is there. They just suddenly pop. The best thing that can happen to a person with an aneurysm is that it is identified incidentally when the patient is having one of several kinds of brain scans for some other reason entirely. The next best thing is for the aneurysm to leak just a little bit of blood, enough to cause symptoms (typically severe headache), but not enough to harm the patient seriously—a so-called "sentinel bleed." Given the opportunity, a neurosurgeon can remove the aneurysm and prevent further bleeding, although it is a risky procedure to have done compared to other surgical operations.

Another cause of bleeding at a single spot in the brain is an arte-
riovenous malformation, or AVM. An AVM is a congenital problem,
meaning that a child is born with the problem. It is an abnormal meshwork of blood vessels, a tangled and interconnected mass of arteries and
veins that is prone to bleed. They come in all sizes and can occur anywhere in the body, although the brain seems to be a relatively common
site for AVMs to occur. They often lie dormant in the brain for years,
even a lifetime, causing no problems until they suddenly bleed. The
severity of the bleeding and the resulting problems are a function of
where and how big the AVM is–little ones in out-of-the-way places may
only cause minor symptoms, big ones in key regions of the brain can
lead to major problems or sudden death when they bleed.

After I had intubated Carrie and given her the mannitol, we
rushed her back down to the CT scanner to find out what had happened so suddenly to her brain. The neurosurgeon went with me to
look at the scan as soon as it was done, since he knew that he might need
to do emergency brain surgery to save Carrie's life and wanted the
answer quickly. As we expected, the CT scan showed new and much
worse bleeding than had been there on Carrie's scan of twelve hours
previously. Judging from the location in the brain, the neurosurgeon sur-
mised that her bleeding was probably from an AVM, not an aneurysm.
At that time the only way to tell for sure what the cause was would have
been to do a test called a cerebral angiogram. This is a high-risk test. It
requires that a radiologist inject the arteries leading into the brain with
a contrast dye that can be seen by a rapid-fire x-ray machine. The x-ray
pictures show where the blood is leaking from the vessels. An angiogram
is high-risk because the test itself can cause a stroke.

At that moment Carrie was deathly ill, at risk of completely her-
niating her brain and dying instantly. All of us–the neurosurgeon, the
neuroradiologist, and me–were afraid that anything that we might do to
perturb her system would kill her, so we did not do the angiogram.
Later, if Carrie survived, we could do the test so that the neurosurgeon
could plan what to do to remove her bleeding source. As we talked, the
nurse called out to me that Carrie's left pupil had again enlarged suddenly, indicating that Carrie was once more on the edge of herniation
and death. Fortunately, her brain once more responded to mannitol and

a few extra breaths on the ventilator, and her pupil reflex returned to normal. We brought Carrie back from the CT scanner to the PICU in the same precarious state. In the elevator, she briefly deteriorated again.

When we got back to her room, the neurosurgeon spoke to Joan about what we could do. The left side of Carrie's brain was extremely swollen and was pushing on her brainstem, the place in the brain where all of our life-sustaining vital functions are located. He told her mother that he believed that Carrie would soon die because he expected the brain swelling to get worse, and Carrie had no leeway for any further pressure inside her head. All that he could offer was to attempt to gain more room for the swelling by removing part of the left temporal lobe of Carrie's brain. This would be a desperate, near-hopeless operation. He told Joan that it might not help even if Carrie survived the operation itself.

Carrie's mother and I sat down at her child's bedside to talk about what to do. She was a highly educated woman with an intrinsic faith in what medical technology could do. Yet she also did not wish to be the one to send her daughter for a dangerous operation, surgery which could kill her, and which might not help anyway. She felt as if this would make her the instrument of her daughter's death. So Joan decided not to do anything except wait, pray, and let us do what we could to reduce the swelling without surgery. I told her that I agreed with her choice. As you read in previous chapters, we doctors often seem to have a bias toward doing something, anything, because it can be a difficult thing just to wait and see what happens. Yet for Carrie, it really was best to watch and wait. Her mother had made the right decision.

We were not completely powerless to help Carrie; there were a few things that we could do. I could continue to give her mannitol and mildly hyperventilate her with the ventilator. More important than what we did do, however, were the things we did *not* do. The brain is a delicate organ, and Carrie had already shown us how sensitive her brain was, how the least little stimulation affected the pressure inside her head. It was therefore vital that we protect her from things that could raise the pressure ever so slightly, things which would normally cause no problem at all, but which in her fragile state could cause her brain to herniate and kill her.

Even when a patient is in a deep, near-death coma such as was Carrie, the brain can react to stimulation from environmental surroundings. For example, I once was transporting a boy in an air ambulance who was nearly as comatose as was Carrie. Before we left, a neurosurgeon had placed a sophisticated, fiber-optic monitoring device in the boy's brain that allowed us to measure minute-to-minute what the pressure actually was. This device allows us to respond quickly to sudden rises in pressure and often prevent the near-herniation events that Carrie was having, events that we could only tell were happening in her brain by examining her eyes. (We use these devices frequently now in these situations, but they were not yet readily available when Carrie was in the PICU.) I was transporting the boy in the middle of winter. It was cold, and we had him well-wrapped in warm blankets. In spite of his deep coma, his brain pressure spiked upward when we opened the door of the ambulance to carry him out to the waiting aircraft, and spiked again when a blast of cold air came through the open aircraft door at our destination. The brain is an astonishingly sensitive organ.

Since Carrie's brain could not stand the least bit of stress, we did all that we could to minimize any stimulation of her senses. We kept her room dimmed and the noise level low. We gave her sedative pain-killing medications. We manipulated her breathing tube and intravenous lines as little as possible. We made sure that her blood oxygen level stayed in a good range, because lack of oxygen, even very briefly, causes a rise in brain pressure. We kept the head of Carrie's bed elevated so that she was partly sitting up and avoided turning her head from side to side, since both of these things help keep the pressure down. After we had done all of these things, paltry measures indeed for such a complex organ as the brain, we waited to see what would happen.

Joan settled in to keep watch at her daughter's bedside. She came from a medical background herself, so she had a good understanding of what everyone had been telling her, particularly of the gravity, even bleakness of the situation. She knew all of that and particularly did not want every doctor and nurse who came through the door to tell her again how hopeless everything looked. She and I quickly reached an understanding: I would be there with her and Carrie for as long as it took for matters to declare themselves, and I would tell her if I thought that anything had changed, but I would not bother her with details of transient ups and downs. Joan mostly sat at Carrie's bedside and read a book.

Doctors and nurses, like everyone, get sick, and so do their families. Caring for a child whose parents are medically astute can be particularly challenging. Parents who are doctors, for example, often ask quite detailed and technical questions about what is going on with their child, and their child's doctors typically answer these questions in a technical fashion–speaking doctor to doctor, as they would to a colleague. Such a professional understanding of the situation might seem to be a useful thing for a parent to have, but this is not always so. Sometimes it even leads to problems.

For one thing, medical practice and medical knowledge have both mushroomed over the past several decades. New medical specialties and subspecialties are appearing all of the time as needs and circumstances change. Pediatric critical care is itself an example of this process; it is barely twenty years old as a formal specialty. This means that, although most medically-knowledgeable parents whose child comes into the PICU know more than the average parent does about what is going on with their child, they may not know as much as they think that they do. We have an expression for that situation: they may know "just enough to be dangerous."

It is a cliché in medicine that doctors and their families sometimes get worse care than do non-medical persons. One reason for this is that the doctors and nurses taking care of them make assumptions about what the family knows or wants to know. The child's caregivers may be afraid of giving offense by being disrespectful of the parents' medical background, but can paradoxically end up not giving the family information that they need and want. The lesson here is that medically-trained parents, like any other parents, should not hesitate to ask about what is going on and why.

Another reason that doctor's families may get substandard care is when the doctor-parent decides to diagnose and treat his or her own child's illness. This is generally not a problem for minor things–sore throats and ear aches–but it can cause serious problems for major illnesses or injuries. It is nearly impossible to exercise good medical judgment when dealing with one's own family, so physician-parents should place their children in the hands of their colleagues.

It is ultimately unfair to ask a doctor or nurse to function in their professional role when their child is sick; they must be allowed, sometimes even gently compelled, to be a parent and only a parent. Their sick child in the PICU already has a flock of doctors and nurses; what the child really needs are parents, and no one can be a doctor or nurse and a parent at the same time.

Carrie had suffered her catastrophic deterioration early in the morning after her admission to the PICU. By noon we knew what had happened and had decided what to do, or not to do. Now all that remained was to wait—the same watchful waiting and supportive care that we gave Tiffany in chapter three. This time, however, none of the PICU staff, myself included, thought that Carrie would survive.

It was difficult to tell what Joan expected. I was in and out of Carrie's room frequently during the afternoon and evening, and her mother never said much about what was on her mind; she mostly sat by the bed and read her book. A friend brought dinner from a local restaurant and the two of them ate it without speaking very much. When it got late, the friend left and Joan dozed in the reclining chair. She slept most of the night, despite the nearly constant, but quiet traffic to and from Carrie's bedside.

I cannot be sure, but I think that Joan was struggling with a set of feelings that trouble any medically-trained person when their child is critically ill. We know the possibilities, the terrible things that can happen suddenly, yet we try to put that knowledge aside and think as any other parent would, be as hopeful as any other parent would be. Joan was also, I believe, struggling with the special variety of guilt that medically-trained parents often feel—that they could have anticipated or even prevented their child's problem. Remember from the first chapter that every PICU parent seems to experience a measure of guilt about what they might have done to prevent their child's illness or injury. This is normal. Medical parents, however, will often wonder why, with their special knowledge, they could not see the problem coming. Carrie most likely had an AVM, something with which she was born. Carrie had, like all children, sometimes complained of a headache and a sore neck: Was either evidence of a small sentinel bleed that might have led to an early diagnosis and safe removal of the AVM? Could Joan, if she had been vigilant, spared Carrie what had happened?

Throughout the night Carrie had several more near-death experiences when spikes of increased pressure in her brain caused her pupil to enlarge and lose its response to light, and her heart rate slowed down. When these happened I would give her additional doses of mannitol and thiopental, a sedative that can briefly lower the pressure, and would give her a few extra breaths on the ventilator. In all of these instances her ominous findings subsided over fifteen to thirty minutes, although truthfully it was impossible to tell if my therapies had anything to do at all with her waxing and waning course. As each one of these episodes occurred, Carrie's nurse would call me into the child's room; each time that I went in there, I expected that I would find that she had herniated her brain and died. But she made it through the night.

The next day Carrie was much the same. This was, in fact, the only faint ray of hope that we had, because brain swelling tends to worsen over the twenty-four hours or so following an event such as Carrie had suffered. So the fact that she was still alive was amazing in itself because, inside Carrie's skull, things were as tight as they could possibly be. When the neurosurgeon came by the PICU to see her at mid-morning, he was astonished to find her still unchanged and alive, particularly when I told him about the spells of increased pressure that she had experienced overnight.

We were both curious about whether her brain swelling had improved, but the only way to tell would have been to send her down for another CT scan. We both agreed that would be dangerous. It also would be wrong because we would not treat her any differently no matter what the scan showed. So even though we were curious, doing the test would have caused serious risk, but provided no potential benefit. As you read in chapter one, parents should always ask this question of their child's doctors: does the potential benefit of the test outweigh the risk (if any) of doing it?

Joan, too, was much the same. She had not slept well in the chair, but she had gotten some rest. Both the neurosurgeon and I spoke with her, and both of us continued to tell her that, in our opinion, Carrie's chances of survival were remote. Still, I did tell Joan that the fact that

Carrie had survived thus far offered a bit of hope because we expected
that the child's brain swelling was likely at its worst. I often tell parents
that before a child can get better, she needs to stop getting worse, and
Carrie appeared to have accomplished that at least. Left unsaid was the
fact that even if Carrie were to live through this, it was unlikely that she
would recover all or even some of her normal brain function; she would
most likely suffer severe and permanent damage. She might even remain
in a persistent vegetative state, like Victoria in chapter eight, forever comatose and dependent upon her ventilator to stay alive.

After the neurosurgeon had left, Joan told me that she appreciated
what she called my optimism. At the time, this seemed to me to be an
unusual thing to say. After all, I had just told her that I still believed that
it was highly likely that her daughter would die. At first I thought that
Joan was being ironic with her comment, since irony is a psychic defense
mechanism that medically-trained persons often use in dire circumstances like this. It can be the mental crutch that we use to get through
difficult situations. The neurosurgeon, who was far more experienced in
this sort of thing than I then was, had told Joan that Carrie would certainly die—if not that day, then definitely the next. I had not painted such
a bleak picture. I am sure that, to the neurosurgeon, this simply showed
how young and inexperienced I was, although he did not say so outright. Perhaps Joan thought the same thing. Still, after I had thought
about it, I realized that she was honestly grateful to me for not taking
away all of her hope.

Joan herself still said little unless I or one of the nurses asked her a
direct question. She had no questions herself. Although she had gotten
some sleep the night before, she was by now showing some of the strain
of twenty-four hours of constant crisis. Carrie's nurse suggested that
Joan might feel better if she left the PICU at least long enough to eat a
meal, shower, and change clothes. The nurse promised that we would
page her immediately if anything at all changed with Carrie. Joan did
not want to leave the hospital, but she did agree to go down and eat
lunch in the hospital cafeteria. After that she went to the hospital staff
locker facility, showered, and came back to the PICU dressed in blue
surgical scrub clothes, making it clear that Joan would not leave the hospital until this was all over.

Even though Joan was unwilling to take a break from her vigil at her daughter's bedside, she did call several of her friends for support. That afternoon a few of them came to visit her and Carrie in the PICU. Many of these friends were also medically-trained—one was a physician who, although she worked in the same facility, practiced a medical specialty that had little to do with pediatric critical care. She told me that she had to go to the main hospital information desk just to find out where the PICU was. All of them sat together with Joan in Carrie's room.

That afternoon turned out to be an eventful one for Carrie. She had only one brief episode of near-herniation, and it was far milder than her previous ones had been. That was good. However, she suffered several other complications of the sort that can bedevil and frustrate the care of critically ill children in the PICU. I spent most of the afternoon and early evening in Carrie's room dealing with these things and trying to fix them.

The first problem was with Carrie's intravenous lines. Her most important one, the one that went into her central venous circulation, malfunctioned. This line was an important part of her care, since we were using it to give Carrie several medications, drugs which supported her heart, her kidneys, and treated her brain swelling. I really did not know if these drugs were actually doing much good, but I did know that it would be a bad time to stop them abruptly, particularly since Carrie's situation appeared to have stabilized a bit.

Soon after three of Joan's friends arrived to visit, Carrie's nurse came to tell me that one of the two central line lumens, the passages within the foot-long device that reached from Carrie's skin into the large central vein above her heart, had clogged. This happens sometimes, and it is usually because a small amount of blood has clotted within the lumen, blocking the flow of drugs and intravenous fluids. It is essentially a plumbing problem, and much as a plumber does with a clogged pipe, we tried several standard tricks to remove the blockage and open the line. None of them worked. Worse, the second of the two lumens also soon quit working. This represented a small crisis because we needed to give Carrie her fluids and medications. Fortunately, Carrie also had an intravenous line in her hand left over from her initial emergency department stay that still worked, and we connected all of her drug infusions to that small catheter, hoping that it could stand the increased flow of all of the fluids until we could get central venous access back.

Joan and her friends watched all of this without saying much, since all of them well understood what was going on and what we needed to do. But when the second lumen clotted off, one of her friends, a nurse with long experience working in an adult intensive care unit, could not help herself; she started to give advice on fixing things, suggestions which became progressively more insistent in tone. She meant well, knowing the risk to Carrie of not keeping good intravenous access, but the tension level in Carrie's room steadily rose. I was very concerned that all of the commotion would cause Carrie's brain pressure to rise, but thankfully that did not happen.

Since I could not unclog Carrie's non-functioning central venous line, I needed to replace it. There is a standard, usually simple way to do this. It is less risky than placing an entirely new line in a different place, which would involve sticking a long needle into the child to search for the central vein. Sometimes this process, which is essentially blind, can result in the needle going astray, perhaps into the child's lung. It is safer instead to pass a fine, flexible wire down one of the malfunctioning lumens until it passes the obstruction and goes out the end of the catheter into the central vein. One can then pull out the old catheter, leaving the wire in place, and slide a new one down the guide wire and back into the vein. Once the new catheter is safely in, the wire comes out, and the problem is solved. It is a simple procedure that we do frequently.

That afternoon nothing was simple for Carrie. Initially her catheter replacement went fine. The guide wire slipped down the old catheter eas-ily, I pulled it out, and I slid a new catheter down the wire. But when I went to the last step, pulling the wire out of the new catheter, the wire would not come out. I tugged on it as firmly as I dared, but it was stuck in the lumen of the new catheter. I had no choice but to pull everything out and start over with a new line at a new site. Once I had pulled it all out, I could see what had happened; there was a small burr, a tiny imperfection on the end of the wire, that had snagged itself and stuck fast in the tip of the catheter. These things happen now and then, but it was especially bad luck for a deathly-ill patient like Carrie. All of this raised the tension in the room even higher, especially when Joan's nurse friend declared that she had never seen such a thing in all of her years working in the intensive care unit. She did not say that it was somehow my fault, but the implication was there.

Although I had confidence in what I was doing and in my technical proficiency, by this time I was getting a bit unsettled by the situation, and I was afraid that it showed. After all, it was very early in my career as an intensivist, and I was working in front of people very knowledgeable in how these procedures were done. As I went out of Carrie's room to get supplies for the new central line that I would need to place, I even considered who I would call if I could not get the line in, even though that is no real disgrace because it happens to all of us from time to time. Carrie's nurse, a woman with many years of experience, followed me out. I remember the scene well. She sat me down in a chair, got me a glass of water, looked straight at me, and said: "You can do this. I've seen you." She was right; I got Carrie's new line in without incident.

If you are a parent in the PICU and find yourself watching this sort of thing happen, you should know that the more complicated the technology, the more likely it is that something will malfunction. These things happen, and although they are frustrating, they are rarely anyone's fault.

The central line was not the only problem that Carrie had that day. Late in the evening, without any warning at all, Carrie began to bleed again. This time it was not in her brain; that would have killed her. This time her bleeding was from her stomach lining, so-called "stress bleeding," a complication which is not uncommon in critically ill patients, especially those with severe head injuries. We use a medication to reduce the chances of this happening, but sometimes it does anyway. Like all the patients whom you have read about on a mechanical ventilator, Carrie had a tube that went through one of her nostrils down to her stomach, a device which she needed to prevent her stomach from becoming bloated with air. Suddenly this tube was filled with fresh blood, and more fresh blood poured from the tube when we connected a suction device to empty her stomach. Carrie kept bleeding for over an hour, even though we kept washing her stomach with iced, clear fluid. She bled so much that I gave her a large blood transfusion. Yet by midnight the bleeding had stopped. Amazingly, or miraculously, Carrie's brain tolerated all of this fine. In fact, she had not had any more near-herniation episodes since early that afternoon.

Joan slept better that night in the reclining chair, although she still had little to say and no questions for me the next morning. The neurosurgeon came to see Carrie and was surprised to find the child still alive, particularly after her episode of stomach bleeding, and he said so to Joan. Several of Joan's friends visited that afternoon, including the physician friend who had been in the PICU the previous day. As it happened, this friend knew the neurosurgeon and had eaten lunch with him that day in the hospital cafeteria. He told her that Carrie's chances of surviving were nil.

Joan's friends stayed in the PICU until late in the afternoon. Her physician friend, the one who had eaten lunch with the neurosurgeon, stopped in to see me where I was working in the physician's office adjacent to the PICU. She stepped into the office and closed the door. She then asked me to tell her exactly what was going on with Carrie. She wanted to know her current medical situation and her chances of surviving in what she termed "any meaningful way." She told me what her opinion was: that the situation was hopeless, that my continuing to "torture" Carrie in the PICU was unethical, and that I was being unfair, even cruel to Joan by not strongly advising her to allow us to take Carrie off life support. She said that, although she herself was no expert in these things, her friend the neurosurgeon was an expert, and he thought that Carrie should be allowed to die.

After she had finished, I asked her whether Joan had told her anything about what she wanted for Carrie. The friend answered that Joan had not told her any specifics. In fact, what would happen to Carrie was a kind of taboo topic among the group, one vaguely alluded to but not really discussed in any direct way. I asked if Joan knew that we were speaking together; the friend answered that she did not. I told her that I believed it was inappropriate for me to tell her anything beyond what I had discussed with Joan that afternoon in Carrie's room, a discussion at which the friend had been present. Confidentiality is doubly important when friends and family work at the medical facility. After all, folks do talk in the cafeteria. I also pointed out to Joan's friend that the neurosurgeon had predicted that Carrie would be dead by now, and that prediction had not proved true. Perhaps he was wrong in other ways.

Joan had thus far been unwilling, or perhaps unable, to talk to me about what she really was feeling and what she wanted for Carrie. I suspected that some of her reticence derived from her medical training; she was not really allowing herself to be a parent, to be Carrie's mother, and not her doctor or nurse. I had not pressed Joan on that issue. After my encounter with her friend, however, I realized that I needed to sit down with Joan and try to have that conversation, if she would allow it.

Late that night I was able to talk to Joan at Carrie's bedside for an hour or so. As we talked, it was clear that, although Joan had been less forthcoming in our discussions than many PICU parents are, we actually understood each other's viewpoint quite well. In fact, that was why she did not feel compelled to elaborate too much during our bedside talks–there was no need. She was actually relieved that I had not pestered her constantly with questions about how she was feeling and what she was thinking. I found this to be a revelation. I had been worried that my relative inexperience as an intensivist made me poorly equipped to provide what she needed in this tragic situation; this was completely untrue. What she appreciated most was that I was there, that I came in to see Carrie frequently, even when I had nothing new to say or a new treatment or test to offer–I was always there.

Early the next morning I was sleeping on a cot in the physician's office when one of the PICU nurses banged on the door to wake me up. She told me that Carrie's nurse wanted to see me immediately. I went into Carrie's room, expecting the worst. "Why now?" I was thinking, "she had been so stable for over twenty-four hours." When I came into the room Joan and Carrie's nurse were standing at the child's bedside. Joan was holding her daughter's hand; when Joan squeezed it, Carrie squeezed back. They were ecstatic. I was excited too, but I well knew that a simple response like that was a long way from Carrie recovering full consciousness. Joan, of course, knew that very well herself–I did not need to tell her, and I did not. Still, it was a start.

Over the next day Carrie awakened even more. She moved her arms and legs when we touched them. By the evening she was taking breaths on her own, even though the ventilator still did most of her breathing for her. All of her normal reflexes had returned by midnight. I began to lighten the doses of sedatives, allowing Carrie to do more and more of her own breathing. Two mornings later I went into her room and called out to her by name; she opened her eyes and looked straight at me. The next morning I pulled out her breathing tube because she was completely awake.

Carrie still had a long way to go in her recovery, of course. Her injury had mostly been on the left side of her brain, near the area where most of us have our speech and language centers. Carrie did have some problems speaking more than a few words at a time, although she appeared to understand what was said to her just fine. She also had some weakness in her right arm and leg. This did not surprise us either; the nerve fibers cross and change sides as they pass down the nervous system, so the right side of the body is controlled by the left side of the brain.

After another week in the PICU, I sent Carrie to another part of the hospital, the rehabilitation unit, where she could get intensive therapy for her speech and motor problems. As it happened, she continued to improve on her own even without the therapy. About a month later, she went home. Before she left, she stopped by the PICU to say goodbye; her arm and leg had returned to normal, and except for an extremely slight hesitancy of speech, something that one would ordinarily not even notice, her speech was entirely normal. She would still need surgery in the near future to have her AVM removed, and the neurosurgeon who had given up on Carrie's survival was delighted to have been proven wrong and to have the opportunity to prevent Carrie from ever again having any bleeding there. He successfully removed the AVM several months later.

I have not heard from Carrie for twenty years and I have no idea where she is and what she is doing. I hope that she is well, because, even though I have cared for thousands of children since, she and Joan taught me lessons that have stayed with me for over two decades; now you know these lessons, too. Even though I may know a great deal, I never really know how things will turn out, so I should be very careful in my predictions. Even when I have nothing to offer but my presence, just being there has value of its own. Finally, I must never take away parents' hope that their child will recover, because although I may know that a child's chances are very, very low, they are never zero. Every once in a while miracles actually happen.

CRITICAL ADVICE FOR PARENTS

No matter how much you know about medicine and your child's problem, you still need to ask questions and make sure that your child's doctor explains things to you.

Tell your child's doctors how much detail in which you would like to receive information; some parents want more, some less—both are perfectly fine.

Expect and accept that malfunctions of PICU technology will happen, especially if your child needs a great deal of it; this is usually nobody's fault.

Try to accept what is truly inevitable, but also never stop hoping for a miracle–doctors are sometimes wrong, and we hope for miracles, too.

Index